School Hardening

Sensory Integration Strategies for Class and Home

Lynne Courtney Tupper, M.P.H., OTR
and
Kathryn E. Klosterman Miesner, OTR

Illustrations drawn under contract by
Cathie Lowmiller

Therapy Skill Builders *®
a division of
The Psychological Corporation

555 Academic Court
San Antonio, Texas 78204-2498
1-800-228-0752

Text copyright © 1995 by Lynne C. Tupper
and Kathryn E. Klosterman Miesner

Illustrations copyright © 1995 by Therapy Skill Builders,
a division of the Psychological Corporation

Published by
Therapy
Skill Builders ®
a division of
The Psychological Corporation
555 Academic Court
San Antonio, Texas 78204-2498
1-800-228-0752

Printed in the United States of America

ISBN 0761643311

10 9 8

Please visit our Web site at www.PsychCorp.com. Please
go to www.psychcorp.com/catg/pdf/survey.pdf to comment on
this or any of our products. Your feedback is important to us.

About the Authors

Lynne Courtney Tupper is a graduate of Rice University and holds a master's degree in Health Services Administration from the University of Texas School of Public Health. Her work experience includes six years with the Texas Department of Human Resources.

When her 5-year-old son was referred for an occupational therapy evaluation due to problems with learning and behavior, Lynne was confused about the role of occupational therapy with children. Over the course of her son's therapy, she came to understand that the occupation of a child is to learn and to play. The positive changes she observed in her son compelled her to change career fields. In 1985 she received the master's degree in Occupational Therapy from Texas Woman's University; and upon graduation, she joined the private practice where her son had received his therapy.

Lynne Tupper is certified in the administration and interpretation of the Sensory Integration and Praxis Tests and is a board-certified pediatric occupational therapist. Currently she serves as clinical director of the Occupational Therapy Center. She lives in Houston with her husband, Robert, and sons David and Robert.

Kathryn E. Klosterman Miesner credits her parents' positive influence in directing her career choices. Her father, a family physician, led the way for her to enter a medical-related field; and her mother, a teacher, talked about how difficult it was for some of her students to learn. A career in occupational therapy has blended both influences.

Kathy is a graduate of the University of Missouri-Columbia. She was originally certified in sensory integration in 1980. Her clinical experience has included coordinating a birth-to-age-three program for Easter Seals in central Illinois; working with children with head injury; traveling as an itinerant therapist in the Houston area public schools; and hospital acute care and rehabilitation in Montana. From 1986 through 1992 she worked in a private practice in Houston, specializing in working with children who have sensorimotor problems. In 1992 she received board certification in Pediatrics from the American Occupational Therapy Association. Currently she is on extended maternity leave, being a full-time mother to Ella, Emilie, and Theodore. Kathy, her husband Tom, and their three children make their home in Katy, Texas.

Contents

Overview

Chapter 1. **School Hardening**—An introduction to the role of occupational therapy for children with learning disabilities

Chapter 2. **Sensory Systems**—An overview of the sensory systems which affect a child's learning potential

Chapter 3. **Motor Planning**—A discussion of the role of praxis, or motor planning, in a child's performance and behavior

Chapter 4. **Evaluation Tools**—A review of standardized evaluations and clinical observations for school-based and private therapists

Chapter 5. **Treatment Ideas**—A collection of treatment activities arranged according to sensory systems

Chapter 6. **Consultation**—An example of how school-based therapists, private therapists, teachers, parents, physicians, and schools can work together

Chapter 7. **Case Studies**—In-depth studies of actual clinical cases, including presenting problems, evaluation results, treatment activities, and outcomes

Preface

Part of the joy in writing this book has been the opportunity to think back over our more than 20 collective years of working with children with special needs. We would like to take this opportunity to offer our thanks to the people who have touched our lives and challenged us to learn more, think more, and pass our knowledge on to others.

Thanks to all the children and their caring, concerned parents who have helped us learn so much about how to help other children. Sharing their frustrations, pain, triumphs, and joys has been a remarkable experience. They have helped us carry our knowledge out of the lecture room and into the clinic where miracles, big and small, happen every day. It is a privilege to be a part of the process.

The clinical stories we have included in this book encompass children from many states and span many years. All of the names have been changed. The stories are told to demonstrate how positive, creative, enthusiastic, and caring people can help make a very real difference in a child's life.

The desire to write this book came out of an experience we shared while presenting at the International Conference on Learning Disabilities in Chicago in 1991. The conference was aimed at providing a place for all interested professionals to share their knowledge and experience in working with individuals with learning differences. There were two primary tracks: medical and educational. For four days, we watched teachers go to the educational sessions and physicians go to the medical lectures. It is time for these tracks to cross. Teachers need to learn what research is being done and how children can be helped with appropriate medical intervention. Physicians need to see the frustration and confusion experienced by teachers as they handle the challenging child on a daily basis in a busy classroom.

This book has not been written exclusively for parents, teachers, or health professionals. The information is intended to encourage dialogue. Each of us has an area of expertise. Listening to one another expands our knowledge base and creates new opportunities for facilitating success. Our children deserve the best that all of us have to offer.

Despite their many similarities, all children are different. They grow and develop and learn in different ways. We must continue to learn about their differences and to explore new avenues to help each child reach the fullest potential.

We also wish to thank the many professionals who have contributed to our knowledge through their writing, presentations, and willingness to serve as our mentors.

Therapists receive extensive instruction about the nervous system as part of their basic training. Continuing education increases that fundamental understanding. Thanks to many dedicated professionals, knowledge continues to be shared and presented in such a way that understanding increases. Some of these professionals include Winnie Dunn, Margot C. Heiniger, Josephine Moore, Shirley Randolph, Orlando L. Schrager, Larry Silver, and Patricia Wilbarger. These professionals are specifically listed because their knowledge and teachings have greatly influenced the writing of this work. Others include Lorna Jean King, Jane Koomar, Shelly Lane, Elizabeth Newcomer, Virginia Scardina, and Patricia Oetter, whose lectures and workshops have contributed to our professional knowledge and enhanced our clinical skills.

And a special thanks to Marietta Maxey, OTR, our mentor and friend, whose work challenged us to follow in her footsteps. It is to her memory that we dedicate this book.

CHAPTER 1

School Hardening

This book is intended as a resource for those who work with school-age children. Teachers and parents frequently are able to identify a discrepancy between a child's apparent potential and actual performance. These discrepancies may play themselves out at home and at school, often affecting behavior as well as learning. Occupational and physical therapists who are experienced in advanced evaluation and treatment techniques may be able to identify and provide appropriate intervention for these children. Although this book is written primarily from the perspective of occupational therapy, it is intended to be collaborative in nature.

In the 1990s, occupational therapy as a profession has taken a turn reminiscent of its historical roots. The concept of *work hardening* refers to the process of reintroducing a patient to the workplace. The process of *work hardening* begins with identifying the barriers to an individual's ability to work. The therapist then provides as much remediation as possible to the person who has an identified disability.

The second phase of the process may include working with the individual to select appropriate adaptations needed to perform specific job tasks. Once that person has achieved the highest possible level of performance, the focus of intervention shifts from the individual to the environment. It becomes incumbent on the workplace to make reasonable accommodations necessary for the potential employee to do the job assigned. The therapist may continue to serve as a consultant to both the employee and employer until the goals are accomplished.

A similar process occurs with children, for whom the appropriate occupation is learning. The accepted workplace for academic learning is school. It is the responsibility of occupational therapists who work with school-age children to assist the child in *school hardening*.

Occupational therapy intervention for children with learning disabilities must include all of the components required for successful school performance. The therapist must identify the barriers to successful learning, initiate a remediation program, assist the child to adapt to the school environment, and work with the child in the school setting to assure that optimal performance is achieved.

The therapist in an adult setting may become even more effective by moving into the workplace, consulting on issues that affect all the workers in a given setting. The therapist may be asked by the employer to assess sitting arrangements, including work height or placement of computer monitors. Important factors affecting performance may include adequate ventilation and lighting. Proper scheduling of break times may enhance individual performance and productivity as a whole.

Similarly, a therapist in a school setting may be called upon to evaluate the learning environment. Not only a child with identified disabilities but all children are affected by the school setting, especially the individual classroom. The occupational therapist may help teachers and administrators to identify environmental factors which affect learning. By tradition and training, a therapist is qualified to assess the effect of sensory stimuli, including noise and other distractions in the classroom. An occupational therapist in the school setting may suggest changes that enhance learning, such as alternative seating arrangements.

Often, parents and teachers are the first to recognize children who do not appear to be performing to their fullest potential. Diagnosticians and special educators can provide valuable information on the child's actual potential and may be able to identify specific areas in which a child needs help. Family physicians and pediatricians can monitor a child's developmental milestones and recommend neurological evaluation when it is indicated. Neurologists can identify structural abnormalities in the brain, identify seizure activity, and confirm subtle deficits in brain function.

Occupational and physical therapists can evaluate functional deficits in a child's performance and provide an appropriate treatment program for the identified deficits. Speech-language pathologists assess the child's ability to use and understand verbal language. Psychiatrists, psychologists, and psychotherapists can help a child and family cope with the identified deficits. Their intervention may help to minimize the adverse affects these conditions may have on a child's psychosocial development. Each professional discipline carries with it a set of assumptions derived from its own historical perspective. These assumptions determine, in part, the professional's role in the evaluation and remediation process.

A child's occupation is to learn, play, and socialize. Rarely do children with learning and attention difficulties have problems only in their academic skills. Associated speech delays may hinder socialization. Delayed gross motor skills will decrease a child's ability to play on the playground, thereby limiting opportunities for appropriate peer interaction. The occupational therapist frequently designs therapy plans to include these aspects of a child's performance.

In the present system of identifying children at risk, it is assumed that a child who is performing adequately in academics is not an appropriate candidate for intervention. Our experience has shown that some of the children performing "within accepted ranges" in school are actually performing much below their cognitive potential. It is only because they are academically gifted that they are able to compensate for underlying deficits in gross or fine motor skills, ability to concentrate, or organizational abilities. Consequently, they have to work extremely hard to keep up with their "average" peers despite their "above average" intellect. Over time, these children seem to become discouraged and may show signs of low self-esteem. They may come to identify themselves as stupid or slow, and they may develop defense mechanisms to protect themselves from failure. While these defensive behaviors may be adaptive in the short run, they may become maladaptive over time.

Popular literature frequently alludes to a high percentage of individuals with learning disabilities among the prison population. One can speculate that this is also true of the homeless population. It is imperative that we make better use of the tools available for early identification of children at risk for school-related problems. Perhaps if these problems are identified and appropriately addressed in childhood, their adverse effect on individuals and on society as a whole might be significantly reduced.

One focus of this book is to encourage professionals who work with children to view both the child and the environment as appropriate areas for intervention. In a hospital setting, a primary physician is assigned to coordinate each case. Such a team leader is generally not as clearly defined in a school setting. A child may have many case managers all assessing their areas of expertise (parent, classroom teacher, diagnostician, special education teacher, speech-language pathologist, physical therapist, occupational therapist). It is a necessary challenge for all of us to work together to analyze each child in each situation. Each team member is important. *We must all learn to look at the whole child.*

By understanding the neurological components that provide the foundation for learning, one can look at the child and the learning environment from a broader perspective. By broadening the scope of the intervention process, the children with whom we work can be better understood and, therefore, better served.

Case Studies

Donald, a 9-year-old boy in the fourth grade, had been identified by the school diagnostician as a child with a high IQ but poor school performance. Tests performed by the diagnostician identified deficits in visual-motor integration. Donald was referred to tutoring to help him with his handwriting. Tutoring proved unsuccessful in improving the quality of his written work, creating further frustration for Donald and his mother. Eventually, he was brought to a private occupational therapy clinic for further evaluation.

The *Sensory Integration and Praxis Tests* (discussed in chapter 4) suggested mild deficits in motor planning abilities and greater deficits in vestibular processing. An occupational therapy program was initiated to address the identified deficits. Over six months of therapy, Donald showed steady progress in vestibular processing and in the ability to accomplish new motor tasks. Much to his relief, handwriting was not directly included in his treatment plan. One day Donald entered the clinic with unusually positive affect, announcing that he had had "a great spelling test." When asked by the therapist what he had made, he reminded her that he always made 100, but this time he had gotten all of his letters within the lines.

Donald graduated from therapy shortly after that memorable spelling test. In addition to improved handwriting, he showed increased self-confidence and a prognosis of continued success in his school work.

While visiting an elementary school for an Admissions, Review, and Dismissal (ARD) meeting for a child with learning disabilities, an occupational therapist was approached by an obviously harried kindergarten teacher. "You've got to help me," she pleaded. "My entire class is impossible. I think they're all hyperactive. I can't keep them in their seats. I can't begin to teach when the kids are all over the room."

Doubting that 25 hyperactive children had somehow been assembled into one classroom, the therapist accompanied the teacher to her room. The children were indeed all over the room. The ones who were attempting to stay in their desks were slipping out or propping themselves up with their arms as they worked. When asked about the desks, the therapist was told that there were more kindergartners than expected and that this classroom had been furnished with desks intended for third graders. The desks were clearly too big for 5-year-olds.

The therapist explained the principle of 90-90 sitting, where the children were supported so that the hips and knees were at 90 degrees and the feet were flat on the floor. The proper desks were requested that afternoon.

On the therapist's next visit to the school, the teacher thanked her for "saving my life." The children were able to sit properly at their desks and attend to the material presented. Without expending extra effort to stay in their seats, they were free to learn. It seems a simple concept, but one completely unnoticed by an experienced teacher who was trained to teach but not to evaluate the physical characteristics of the classroom.

These case studies reiterate the importance of a collaborative effort in working with children. In Donald's case, school assistance, parent involvement, and private therapy teamed to facilitate his ability to work in the school environment. Classroom consultations also have an important place, as shown in the second illustration.

Just as the process of work hardening in the rehabilitation setting helps a patient eliminate the barriers to returning to an occupation or work, school hardening must do the same for the school-age child. *School Hardening* represents a collaborative effort among child, parents, teaching professionals, school staff, allied health professionals, and medical professionals to assess each child and situation. The goal is to create an environment for the child to perform successfully. Academic learning as well as physical, social, and emotional factors need to be considered to make the school environment a place where the child can succeed.

CHAPTER 2

Sensory Systems

This chapter will review portions of the sensory nervous system with specific emphasis on learning. Everyone knows that the five basic senses provide our nervous systems with information about vision, hearing, smelling, tasting, and touching. However, there are other parts of the nervous system not as well recognized which also contribute to the ability to learn.

The nervous system needs information from many receptors to form an accurate assessment of the environment. When one part of the system is not functioning, the central nervous system does not receive a complete picture. For example, if a child is hearing impaired, that child's perception of the world is different from that of a child with normal hearing. When the child receives hearing aids, the perception of the world changes. This change increases the child's ability to interact effectively in the environment.

Many children who experience difficulties in school (especially those with no clearly defined medical diagnosis or etiology) appear to be receiving incomplete sensory information and consequently are not able to respond appropriately to the demands of the school environment. As sensory systems are discussed, consider the following case studies involving John, Matthew, and Laura.

John, age 12, had been placed in a private school after repeated incidents of behavior problems in his local public school. John's parents felt that a smaller school with a more nurturing environment would decrease John's acting-out behaviors. However, behavior problems continued to occur in the new school. His teachers noted that he became uncomfortable in groups, preferred to be the last in the line, refused to sit in the front of the classroom, and insisted on wearing his jacket (not a part of the school uniform) despite warm weather. His teacher stated, "I am so busy dealing with his idiosyncrasies, I'm embarrassed to say I'm not sure if he is learning anything!"

Matthew, age 9, was sent for private occupational therapy testing as a last resort. His mother, in tears, reported that he used to be nice to his sister, loved to go to school, and played quietly. Recently, he had been involved in fights at school, kicked his sister so hard her leg was broken, and hit his mother in frustration while doing handwriting homework. His grades were adequate, although his teachers complained of slow, poor handwriting.

Laura, age 4, had a medical diagnosis of developmental delay. Generally she was quiet, withdrawn, and preferred to sit and watch TV, play by herself, or be held. Her mother reported that Laura screamed in terror the one time she attempted to swing her. Laura had much difficulty stepping over curbs. She refused to climb. In the bathtub, she persistently refused to allow her mother to wash her hair.

All of these children were experiencing difficulties with reception, perception, or processing of sensory information. It was affecting the lives of their families and their ability to learn in school and socialize with peers.

A simplified explanation of the neurology of the tactile, proprioceptive, kinesthetic, and vestibular systems follows.

Tactile System

The tactile system is the first part of the nervous system to begin to function in utero. At the six-week gestational age, the fetus will move in response to touch. It is reportedly the most mature system at birth. The rooting response is a response to tactile input. When an infant's cheek is lightly touched, the infant will turn to that side to "root" for a nipple. Research has shown that infants who receive much tactile input (touching and holding) gain weight faster than those not receiving as much tactile input (Cochran 1986).

Neurologically there are two basic types of tracts (pathways in the spinal cord that transmit information) dealing with touch sensations. They are the *spinothalamic tract* and the *lemniscal tract*. These tracts carry the touch information up the spinal cord to the sensory areas in the cerebral hemispheres.

The spinothalamic tract is more primitive and is the primary tactile tract functioning at birth. Its characteristics include these:

- It warns of danger.
- It causes the nervous system to prepare for fighting or fleeing (commonly called the "fight or flight" response).
- It responds to less specific touch such as hair displacement on the arm, or light, brushing touch.
- It may trigger the body to feel afraid, like "a pit in the stomach."

The lemniscal system matures more slowly. It has the potential to override the spinothalamic tract or clarify the information sent to the brain by the spinothalamic tract. The lemniscal tract carries more localized and specific information. For example, the spinothalamic tract can warn the nervous system that it was brushed, and the lemniscal tract can contribute that the sensation was soft, warm, and moved slowly. The lemniscal tract could override the initial alert-and-fear response by contributing more information so that the brain could determine that the touch was cloth from a scarf blowing in the wind. Some other characteristics of the lemniscal tract include these:

- It assesses the amount of pressure in a touch.

- It senses movement.

- It can localize the exact spot of a touch.

Dysfunctions in the tactile system can be summarized as being either overly sensitive to touch or overly unresponsive to touch. The somatosensory system allows an individual to sense joint movement and touch sensations. The child with somatosensory processing problems may not be able to feel or localize a tactile stimulus. Conversely, the child with an overresponsive tactile system knows exactly what touched the body, to the point that this child is highly distracted by inadvertent touch from the environment.

Children with poor tactile sensitivity do not have the benefit of feedback as to how they have moved. It's as though their skin is covered with a thick coat.

Benjamin had many symptoms of poor sensory feedback. When he opened the door, he consistently ran it into his foot. As he carried a glass, he was unaware that it was tilting and liquid was penetrating his shirt. While climbing the ladder to the slide, he needed to watch his foot on each step because his leg did not seem to sense how far to lift to reach the next step. Fine motor skills were nearly impossible because he broke his pencils and crayons, tore the paper, and squeezed the glue bottle too hard.

When William received a severe burn, his mother was amazed that he did not cry. He was constantly covered with bruises, but they never seemed to bother him. When he came into class from the playground, often his shoes were filled with sand, but he never seemed to notice.

Both William and Benjamin had tactile systems that did not seem to interpret touch information from their environment.

Tactual defensiveness is the term frequently used to describe the child who is overly sensitive to touch. These children do not seem to have a mature lemniscal tract to override the more primitive spinothalamic tract. The primitive tactile system is alerted by any touch, causing the more discriminative aspects of touch to be ignored or misinterpreted by the nervous system.

Chad could not tolerate a label in his shirt. If he was bumped in the lunch line, he turned with fists ready to fight. He was not able to tolerate walking in crowds. He refused to walk barefooted in the grass or on the carpeting. He wore his socks constantly. His mother commented that he had never let her hug him. All of these "unusual" behaviors have a common denominator of hypersensitivity to tactile stimuli.

Glenna's grandmother loved her very much, but she believed that Glenna hated her. She had bought a beautiful Easter dress which the child refused to wear. In tears, she reported that Glenna had cut up the dress with scissors, trying to cut out the petticoat. The grandmother interpreted the child's behavior as a personal rejection, rather than an indicator of a disordered tactile system.

Wilbarger and Wilbarger (1991) expanded on the concept of tactual defensiveness and identified a set of behaviors which may be termed *sensory defensiveness.* Children (and adults) who are distracted by touch sensations frequently also are adversely affected by visual stimuli, particularly light. They may overreact to sounds and be labeled *auditorily defensive.* Smells may become overwhelming and result in nausea. These symptoms are caused by an overly active sympathetic nervous system and are associated with excess adrenalin. With all of these sensations bombarding the cortex of the brain, it is no wonder that children with this set of responses may be identified as having attention deficits.

Understanding that there are neurological reasons to explain behaviors goes a long way toward identifying and treating the problems. Adults working with these children need to understand why these children act the way they do. Behavior programs are probably not the answer to dysfunctions in the tactile receptors. The case study of John (page 7) is an example of a child with severe tactual defensiveness. By understanding the reasons behind his unusual behaviors, his teachers and parents became more tolerant. John was allowed to be last in line so that he could monitor potential touch problems and keep on his jacket to protect his arms from incidental touch. By providing appropriate intervention to normalize the tactile system, incidents of fights with peers decreased.

Guidelines for Working with a Child Experiencing Tactual Defensiveness

1. Do not pat the child on the back. Unseen touch is especially threatening to the nervous system. Rather than rewarding the child with a pat on the back, approach from the front and make sure the child is aware of your presence before reaching out. Be cognizant of the child's facial expression. It will tell you whether to touch or to *leave the child alone.*

2. Let a tactually defensive child initiate touch. Make yourself available for a hug, but do not impose one on the child. Getting an unwanted hug is not a pleasant experience. Firm or deep-pressure touch is more comforting to a disordered nervous system than light, moving touch. Touch gently but firmly. Bear hugs may be more easily tolerated than "ticklish" touch.

3. Respect differences in clothing preferences. Tactually defensive children often object to "itchy" clothes, labels, and socks with seams. Be patient; over the course of treatment, as defensiveness decreases, the child may be able to tolerate a wider range of textures and clothing. Until the defensiveness lessens, wearing comfortable clothes may decrease distractions and increase the child's attention to task.

4. In a group situation, allow the tactually defensive child to be at the periphery of the group or at the back of the line. This arrangement allows the child more control by having a better opportunity to anticipate touch and fewer possibilities for inadvertent touch.

Children who are overly sensitive to touch also may react to other types of sensory stimuli. Bright lights or loud noises may distress them. Odors may cause nausea. Certain types or textures of food may be unpleasant. It is important to be aware that these responses are the result of disordered sensory systems which are not within the child's control. The child's responses to these sensations may include bossiness or other controlling behaviors. These negative behaviors frequently diminish as sensory processing improves. By respecting the child's nervous system, we can help create a safer, less threatening environment while treatment addresses the source of the problem.

Proprioception

The term *proprioception* refers to the sensations received from the muscles and joints. Proprioceptive input tells the brain when and how the muscles are moving. This information helps the individual know where and how the body is moving without having visual assistance. There are numerous spinal tracts carrying this information to the brain. Much of the information is relayed to the cerebellum. Proprioception, when used in conjunction with tactile awareness and kinesthesia, gives the brain more complete information about the environment. Children with poor proprioception may inadvertently break their toys. These children do not have an accurate sense of how hard they are pushing or pulling a toy. They may appear to be overly rough for the same reasons.

Benjamin (page 10) showed many symptoms of poor proprioception. He was unable to sense how far to lift his foot for placement on stairs. Pencils were broken and glue squeezed too hard for the same reasons.

Lyndsey was holding the therapist's hands while jumping on a mini-trampoline as part of her therapy session. She commented that she could not close her eyes because her legs would not tell her where to jump.

Kinesthesia

The sense of kinesthesia combines proprioception and tactile sensations to provide the brain with information about movement of body parts in relation to each other. Intact kinesthetic sensations are required for throwing balls, playing tennis or golf, climbing stairs, typing, writing, and riding a bike. The body needs sensory clues from its body parts to make continual, subconscious readjustments to the motor performance. For example, if a toe is injured, the body automatically adjusts its standing position.

Matthew (discussed on page 8) is a good example of the importance of kinesthesia. He was evaluated, using the *Sensory Integration and Praxis Tests* (SIPT), discussed further in chapter 4. This evaluation revealed average scores in all areas except kinesthesia. His Kinesthesia score on the SIPT was two standard deviations below the norm. Poor kinesthesia easily explains his difficulties with handwriting. Matthew did not have adequate sensory feedback in his hands to allow him to write without visually monitoring and directing each pencil stroke. Since academically and physically he appeared "normal," there was no apparent "excuse" for his frustration and dislike of handwriting. Information provided by the SIPT alleviated Matthew's parents' frustrations and provided neurological explanations of the problem to his parents and teachers. The kick that broke a bone in his sister's leg is a tragic example of poor sensory feedback as to how much force is being exerted. It also graphically demonstrates the frustrations these children may feel when they are trying to "do better" and can't.

Vestibular System

Perhaps the most misunderstood portion of the nervous system is the vestibular mechanism. The vestibular system is partially responsible for the sense of balance as well as awareness of movements to the head and body. The vestibular system consists of the *semicircular canals, utricle* and *saccule.* They are located in the inner ear and share the eighth cranial nerve with the hearing portions of the ear. Information from the vestibular system is processed primarily in the brainstem. However, many parts of the brain receive vestibular information.

Vestibular information also descends to many areas of the body. The vestibular system plays an integral part in regulating the body's muscle tone, postural reactions, balance, and coordination ocular movements. The semicircular canals are primarily receptive to rolling and rotation. The utricle and saccule respond more to linear acceleration and deceleration and the constant pull of gravity. As gravity is constantly pulling on the utricle and saccule, the central nervous system is constantly being informed about the body and head orientation in space.

Problems with vestibular processing can be summarized by being either overly responsive to stimuli or underresponsive to stimuli. The Postrotary Nystagmus test (part of the *Sensory Integration and Praxis Tests*) is a standardized test designed to evaluate one aspect of vestibular functioning. A therapist must be properly trained to administer this assessment accurately. However, clinical observation alone can provide a tremendous amount of information about a child's vestibular system.

Laura's story (discussed on page 8) is a classic case of an overly sensitive vestibular system. Her response to swinging was one of fear. She had difficulty with the slight up-and-down movement required to negotiate curbs and steps. She had little desire to be mobile; rather, it was much more comfortable for her vestibular system for her to sit, which was not fear provoking. However, because of her vestibular system's oversensitivity to movement, her central nervous system was essentially deprived of vestibular sensory input. Consequently, her muscle tone was poor, she had weak neck and back extensor muscles, and her eye control was poor. Understanding the function of the vestibular system cleared up many questions for her parents. Her teachers also understood why she preferred to lie on the floor or hold her head up with her hands and why she could not seem to focus her eyes. Occupational therapy with an emphasis on normalizing vestibular processing was an integral part of her treatment. The information provided by the evaluation was helpful in defining and explaining the neurological basis for some of her learning difficulties.

Laura's vestibular system was overly sensitive to motion. The term *gravitational insecurity* is used for this type of sensitivity. The words describe how individuals with this condition feel about what gravity is doing to them. The constant pull of gravity is generally experienced in a vertical position (walking, sitting); and when that sensation is changed (for example, by swinging, ascending or descending stairs, or leaning backward), the child experiences a fear or insecurity about how the body will respond to the change in the pull of gravity. This is an emotional response and may produce vertigo, nausea, vomiting, and other physical symptoms. Gravitational insecurity is a very real fear (although it may seem out of proportion to the actual danger of the activity). The child's fear must be respected by the child's therapists, parents, and teachers. A child with gravitational insecurity must never be forced to participate in an activity that will provoke fear.

When a child's vestibular system is underresponsive to motion, the child can roll, turn around, spin, and jump without feeling the sensation of dizziness. Normally, all young children can tolerate motion better than adults. However, some children's nervous systems do not seem to "register" what is occurring in the environment. These children may seem to be constantly on the move.

Recent research by Kimball (1986) has suggested an association between a depressed postrotary nystagmus score and so-called hyperactivity. Her work suggests that children who are labeled hyperactive and have a low postrotary nystagmus score may respond well to drug therapy using Ritalin, a neurostimulant. This group of children also tends to respond favorably to occupational therapy using sensory integrative treatment techniques, including vestibular stimulation.

Six-year-old Nathan's Postrotary Nystagmus score on the SIPT suggested that his nervous system was not processing vestibular information in an average manner. He had a history of chronic ear infections and had recently received his fourth set of pressure-equalizing tubes. One can speculate that vestibular processing was compromised by a chronically infected ear, a malformed inner-ear mechanism, pinching of the auditory-vestibular nerve due to pressure from increased fluid, or central nervous system defects. Regardless of the etiology, the effect was a child with poor extensor muscle tone, poor balance responses, and delayed speech. In school he was described as "hyper," fell out of his chair frequently while concentrating on writing, and had fine motor skills below those of his peers.

When any one of these lesser-known components (tactile, kinesthetic, proprioceptive, vestibular) is not functioning, the information received by the central nervous system is incomplete and, therefore, less accurate.

Summary

The intention of this chapter is primarily to inform the readers of some of the idiosyncrasies associated with inefficient tactile, proprioceptive, and kinesthetic processing. However, clinically, it is often difficult to differentiate problems with proprioception from tactile or kinesthetic problems. The *Sensory Integration and Praxis Tests* (SIPT) contain evaluations designed to assist in differentiating these systems. The SIPT and other evaluation tools are discussed in chapter 4.

See page 110 for suggested readings on sensory integration and sensory systems.

CHAPTER 3

Motor Planning

Motor planning, also termed *praxis,* forms the foundation for motor performance. It may be described as that subconscious sense which allows our bodies to respond to what our brain directs. Before we can accomplish a task, we must be able to comprehend the task and devise a plan to approach and execute it. Deficits in motor planning may explain why a child who understands a concept may be unable to apply the concept to a motor task.

Toward the end of her life, Dr. A. Jean Ayres focused increasingly on praxis as a necessary foundation for learning and classroom performance. In her monograph, *Adult-Onset Apraxia and Developmental Dyspraxia* (Ayres 1985), she wrote, "Praxis is the sense which allows us to interact with the physical world in the way that speech allows us to interact with the human world." Ayres differentiated between motor-planning deficits in adults who had once had planning abilities and lost them through trauma or stroke, and children who had not yet developed these abilities.

Children with poor motor-planning skills may work slowly and inefficiently to accomplish tasks that come more easily to their peers. They may be able to describe a task but not physically perform it. This inconsistency may be frustrating for teachers and parents who can see that the child has adequate understanding but fails to perform. It is easy to assume that the task could be accomplished if only the child would try harder. What is not easy to understand is that children with dyspraxia are trying harder than their peers. However, the increased effort is not reflected in the end product.

Children who lack spontaneous motor planning ability frequently learn to cope by using the thinking and reasoning areas of their brains to compensate for deficits in more automatic motor performance. Such compensation requires increased energy, placing the child at risk for fatigue, frustration, and the development of a poor self-image. These children are frequently described as very hard workers, but they may not have energy left for spontaneous, creative fun. As school tasks become increasingly complex, these children may have difficulty keeping pace with their peers who learn new tasks more efficiently.

Children with dyspraxia typically have a difficult time learning new motor skills. While they may not spontaneously grasp the new motor skills, with practice they can become skillful at specific tasks. These learned skills are called *splinter skills* because they must be learned by repetition. Splinter skills do not tend to generalize to similar tasks.

An example of a splinter skill is evident in Joseph's shoe tying. At age 7, he had finally learned to tie his shoes. One day a friend's shoe came untied, and Joseph offered to tie it for him. However, the shoe was not oriented as he was used to tying, and the laces were longer. Although Joseph could tie his own shoes, the splinter skill did not transfer when the components were slightly altered.

The fact that children with dyspraxia can be taught specific tasks makes it even more difficult to understand the deficits involved. Parents and teachers frequently attempt to teach these children everything they need to know to carry out activities of daily living. For example, they may devise checklists to help a poorly organized child to establish a morning routine of getting up, dressing, and coming to breakfast. Children who come to rely on external mechanisms may have a very difficult time coping with even minor changes in routine. They may resist eating before getting dressed if that is not part of their usual morning routine. They may become frustrated when the new jeans have buttons rather than snaps. Little changes add up to big adjustments for these children.

David, 4 years old, was easily capable of dressing himself for school, including buttoning his shirt. One morning, his mother came to the door of his room and handed him a cowboy shirt with snaps instead of buttons. David struggled with the shirt for a few minutes and finally threw it on the floor and stomped on it. When his mother asked him to explain his behavior, he exclaimed, "The damn buttons are broken." David's story illustrates the frustration often experienced by children with dyspraxia.

In school, these children may be able to follow a routine day of reading, math, lunch, recess, social studies, science, and physical education, but may fall apart if there is a fire drill, a change in schedule, or—worse yet—a substitute teacher. Their inability to adjust to change may result in controlling behaviors designed to force predictability onto people and events which seem perilously unpredictable to them.

Rex was a bright 9-year-old who bragged continuously about his athletic prowess. However, when presented with a new motor task, he attempted to avoid the activity by labeling it "dumb" and "boring." He frequently attempted to manipulate the therapist by changing the activity to a more familiar one or by talking about how well he would do the activity until there was no time left to attempt it.

One hallmark of dyspraxic behavior is reliance on a very narrow repertoire of skills. A child may attempt unsuccessfully to apply old, trustworthy skills to a new situation. Children who stack blocks successfully may attempt to stack miniature cars. If playing with cars is their established skill, they may attempt to play with blocks by lining them up and pushing them around. They are frequently described as perseverative in their behavior, having difficulty letting go of one activity to move on to another one.

Five-year-old Carolyn came to therapy twice a week for 30 minutes. At the beginning of virtually every session, she stated, "I want to draw a picture." The therapist usually attempted to redirect her to a different activity, promising to allow her to draw a picture later. By the time Carolyn was engaged in another activity, she often refused to change to drawing her picture, saying, "Not now. I'm busy."

Praxis plays an important role in the development of speech and language. Oral-motor skills are necessary for adequate articulation. A child with poor praxis may have difficulty placing the tongue in the proper position to produce a specific sound. Children with a limited repertoire of motor skills may show similar limits in their language abilities. Dyspraxic children may use repetitive sentence structure, employ few modifiers, and cling tenaciously to limited subject matter. While these characteristics appear in children with learning disabilities, they are much more clearly manifested in children with pervasive developmental disorders and autism.

Evan was referred for an occupational therapy evaluation by his speech pathologist who felt that poor praxis was significantly limiting his speech and language development. Since he was only 3 years old at the time, evaluation of his praxis was done in a nonstandardized manner, observing his approach and interaction with unfamiliar pieces of therapy equipment. He sat on top of a "Sit-n-Spin" toy rather than on the bottom where he could use the top to make himself spin. He was able to climb up a step, but could not step over an inner tube lying on the floor. These behaviors were interpreted by the therapist as evidence of dyspraxia.

Over the course of his treatment, Evan was presented with various motor activities that encouraged transfers between pieces of suspended equipment. His mother reported that his speech development appeared to mirror his motor-planning skills. For example, when he was able to interact with single pieces of equipment, he used single-word phrases. As he increased his motor repertoire, his speech kept pace. When he began to transfer between pieces of equipment, he began to use two-word phrases. When two transfers occurred at the same time, he began to use three-word phrases; and so on, until he could negotiate a multitransfer obstacle course and speak in complete sentences.

Proper evaluation and treatment for these children is necessary to obtain a better understanding of their weaknesses and frustrations. Looking for common-denominator problems related to poor motor planning may help relieve a parent's frustration. Knowledge and understanding of the problems related to motor planning can lead to appropriate options for remediation. A therapist may provide treatment to enhance motor planning abilities. The therapist also may make suggestions to parents to help the child compensate for the deficiencies and better accommodate to novel motor tasks.

Dr. Ayres (1985) differentiated among three types of motor planning problems: ideational dyspraxia, sequencing or organizational problems, and difficulties with execution.

A child with ideational problems may be unable to formulate a plan of attack for a new activity. This problem may be cognitive in nature and respond appropriately to a cognitive approach to therapy. Such a child may benefit from being "talked through" an activity or by having the appropriate steps modeled by the therapist or another child.

Evan, mentioned above, was an example of a child with ideational dyspraxia. He was frequently able to do an activity when it was modeled for him. For example, he learned to use tools by working with his father in his workshop. Evan could hammer and use a screwdriver, but he was unable to build with blocks until the therapist showed him how.

A child who appears to understand the required task but seems unable to get organized sufficiently to accomplish it may have difficulty with sequencing or organizational skills. This child may require the task to be divided into its component parts before the child can attempt it. Once the plan is made, this child may have little or no trouble with its execution.

Rex had difficulty formulating a plan. The more complex the task, the more he talked. He could frequently describe exactly how to negotiate a suspended obstacle course ("Climb up the ladder, go to the tire swing, and swing onto the log"). But when he attempted to follow his own directions, he was unable to accomplish his plan because he couldn't get organized. This is termed *somatodyspraxia*. Despite adequate motor skills, he had difficulty initiating a new activity, sequencing it appropriately, and following through. His schoolwork reflected the same difficulties.

The third type of praxis problem is one of execution. A child with performance problems may be limited by poor physical development such as abnormal muscle tone or tremor.

Simon had a lot of wonderful ideas about what to do and how to go about it, but he seldom accomplished his goals. He had a seizure disorder that required medication. When the medicine dosage was sufficient to control the seizures, he developed a tremor in his hands, which severely limited his fine motor skills.

In Simon's case, modifications (such as a clipboard to stabilize his paper and wrist weights to increase proprioceptive feedback to his hands) helped him to accomplish his goals. For many children with dyspraxia, appropriate therapy is directed toward expanding their repertoire of skills, which in turn allows them to become more flexible in their interactions with people and things.

Case Studies

Richard, age 4, was brought to an occupational therapist for an evaluation of poor gross motor and fine motor skills. He was administered the *Sensory Integration and Praxis Tests* (see pages 29-30), which clearly supported a diagnosis of dyspraxia. His test scores were likened by the computer-generated chronograph to somatodyspraxia. He had particularly low scores in Postural Praxis and Oral Praxis which required him to imitate movements modeled by the examiner. Richard's case study was published in the *American Journal of Occupational Therapy* (Tupper 1990).

During the parent conference, Richard's father stated emphatically that his son did not have motor-planning problems and was, in fact, extremely well organized. He decided not to seek treatment for the child. The therapist observed the father's interactions with the child as they left the clinic. The child was playing with a basket of toys in the waiting room. The father told him to pick up the toys and get ready to go. "Stop playing now," he said. "It's time to go. Richard, pick up the toys. No, pick them up and put them in the basket. No, Richard, pick up the toys like this, one at a time, and put them in the basket. Richard, listen to me. Watch now. I'm picking up this block and putting it in the basket. Now you pick one up. No, Richard. Are you listening? Pick up the toys and put them in the basket like this. . . ."

Fifteen minutes later, the father had finished picking up the toys and had talked Richard through putting on his jacket. He left the office, still convinced that Richard did not have a praxis problem. Well-meaning parents and teachers may inadvertently impose their own planning and organization abilities onto the child, as if programming a robot, and thereby overlook the child's poor organizational skills. It is unfortunate to see a father working so hard to help his child and, by doing so, missing an opportunity to provide a better kind of help.

Richard's story provides an excellent illustration of the fact that one should not have to verbally cue each step of a task. Because we humans are thinking creatures, we assume there is nothing we can't think through to accomplish. This is true. However, there are many things that we should not have to think through. For most of us, picking up toys, getting dressed, copying written work, and eating do not take our active attention.

However, if the situation changes (say you have a broken arm), all of these normally easy tasks have to be "re-thought." By the end of a day of re-thinking these normally easy tasks, you'd be exhausted.

Although well-meaning teachers and parents are able to create a way for this type of child to manage the day by providing a detailed program of step-by-step directions, one must not overlook the possibility of an underlying sensory processing problem. Unless that underlying sensory processing problem is identified and remediated, the child will have to continue to "think through" rote tasks. By providing appropriate remediation, the child's energy may be redirected to academic learning, creativity, and fun.

Alexander's preschool teacher did not feel he was ready for kindergarten. She suggested Alexander have developmental testing performed to help the parents make a more informed decision about school placement. The diagnostician noted Alexander's dyspraxic tendencies and referred him for a SIPT evaluation. Alexander's standardized SIPT results confirmed the suspicions. His parents were relieved to hear there was a reason behind all of his "annoying" tendencies (knocking over his milk each meal, falling and tripping for no obvious reason, breaking his toys, running into the plant stands, . . .).

Bryan was a bright, articulate 9-year-old with significant behavior problems. He seemed to work very hard, even at things that should have been fun. He appeared to be constantly frustrated and angry. When things didn't go as he had anticipated, he became extremely upset—even violent.

Bryan had broken his nose while playing T-ball at age 7. He later told his mother, "I moved behind the ball like the coach said, but I forgot to put up my glove." He worked hard at written assignments, often writing and erasing so hard that he left holes in his paper. He had difficulty organizing tasks and often appeared clumsy and awkward.

An evaluation by an occupational therapist suggested that he had deficits in praxis. He received treatment for approximately six months, at which time his test scores were age-appropriate and he was discharged from therapy. Following his discharge, Bryan's mother asked him if he could do more things since having therapy. After careful thought, he replied, "No, I don't think I can *do* more things; I just think the things I do are easier and *funner*." For a child who usually showed only frustration and anger and seldom appeared happy or joyful, easier and "funner" led to a significant change in his behavior and in his interactions with others.

Many teachers and parents have been surprised to learn about dyspraxic disabilities in their children because the children appear to have good large-motor skills. Although a child may be good at running, jumping, throwing, or riding a bike, one cannot assume normal motor planning. Vincent is an excellent example. Vincent was attending a private school because his parents felt his neighborhood public school was too large a place for him. They felt he would actually get lost! In second grade, his academic scores were continuing to fall and his behavior was becoming a problem at school and at home. The only thing going right for Vincent was making the All-Star T-ball team in his town. His physician referred him for occupational therapy testing, using the SIPT at Vincent's mother's request.

During the testing, he was not able to balance on one foot for more than two seconds and was unable to walk heel-to-toe. Vincent's complete SIPT scores suggested he had poor touch-discrimination abilities and below-average motor planning. The poor motor-planning scores were very surprising, considering his reported bike-riding and T-ball abilities. Closer examination of his bike-riding habits revealed he always rode the same path in his neighborhood and refused to ride on the dirt bike paths created by his peers. In T-ball, his coach said, "Vincent can't field a ball, but as long as the other team members throw it right to him on first base, he always catches it. I just always have him play first base." Analysis of this situation suggests playing first base required significantly less motor-planning adaptations than shortstop or fielding. Vincent had practiced and was sufficiently motivated to work hard at T-ball. The same was true for bike riding. He desperately wanted to be like his peers and learned to ride a bike, but had to limit his riding to paths he knew which required less motor planning.

Vincent's testing helped explain to his parents and teachers those things he was good at doing and why he resisted things like riding his bike on a new path. During his course of therapy, as his motor planning and motor skills improved he was able to accept more changes in his routine and make appropriate adaptations without displaying inappropriate behavior.

Summary

Motor planning can be puzzling. Each day, our routines utilize many automatic motor plans. For example, brushing teeth requires little cognitive attention; we perform it without thinking. However, if the toothpaste container springs a leak, the routine motor plan needs to be changed. For most of us, this is an adaption easily accomplished. A child with poor ideational motor planning may have no idea how to remedy the situation. A child with poor coordination may know what needs to be done but be unable to coordinate fingers to accomplish the repair.

As long as the routine is going as it should, little motor planning is required. Think again to the challenged child who faces each school day with an unlimited number of potential changes. The dyspraxic child may have many worries about an upcoming day. ("What if the pencil breaks? What if I have a substitute teacher? What if we have to learn a new game in physical education? What if I can't sit in my same seat on the bus?" The list could be endless.) It is important to realize the emotional energy dyspraxic children may be expending without really accomplishing anything for school.

A dyspraxic child may need additional verbal cuing to prepare for the day. Extra time for dressing, breakfast, and school preparation may decrease stress. New activities or changes in routine may require gradual introduction and positive reinforcement. Parents, teachers, and professionals can honor the child's nervous system by permitting harmless routines and idiosyncrasies. Understanding why a child may have certain preferences may go a long way in making the school and home environments sensitive to the needs of the child.

CHAPTER 4

Evaluation Tools

The evaluation process is an integral part of identifying deficits and establishing an appropriate treatment program. While the diagnostician can measure a child's cognitive function and academic potential, the occupational or physical therapist is uniquely qualified to assess the sensorimotor components required for adequate performance in the school setting. This chapter may be of greater interest to therapists, diagnosticians, and teachers who already are familiar with standardized tests. However, parents or others who are less familiar with these specific tests will learn valuable observational skills that are helpful in analyzing a child's strengths and weaknesses.

Many types of evaluations have been developed to measure a child's level of function. Developmental checklists can establish a baseline for the child's gross and fine motor skills as well as social and self-help skills. These scales are simple to administer and have good interrater reliability. They may be administered by any professional or paraprofessional with special training. When an occupational therapist administers a developmental evaluation, important clinical observations may be made. These observations serve to make these instruments useful for both identifying lags and forming a treatment program for remediation.

These clinical observations may include the child's level of attention and activity, overall muscle tone, postural mechanisms, and reflex integration. A child's eye and hand usage can give information on the development of dominance, hemispheric specialization, and bilateral integration. Observing the quality of a child's movement patterns can give the therapist clues as to motor-planning skills and the amount of effort required for the child to accomplish age-appropriate tasks.

Gross and fine motor batteries such as the Bruininks-Oseretsky *Test of Motor Proficiency* (Bruininks 1978) and the *Peabody Developmental Motor Scales* (Folio and Fewell 1983) can help to determine an age-equivalent score for the child's motor performance. These tests are not by nature diagnostic, but they can be used to establish a baseline against which to measure change over time.

The comparison of similar tests may be useful in determining the major areas of a child's deficits. For instance, the *Developmental Test of Visual-Motor Integration* (Beery and Buktenica 1989) may show that a child's visual-motor performance is below age expectation, but it does not specify which component is the underlying cause of the lag. A child may perform poorly due to a vision problem. This possibility may be assessed by school or medical testing. Another source of difficulty may be visual-perceptual deficits. These may be identified by administering a nonmotor test of visual perception. If these two areas are ruled out as problem areas, the therapist may look further at the motor component of a child's performance.

During a child's performance on a visual-motor test, an experienced therapist notes handedness, pencil grasp, and how much pressure the child uses to move the pencil. The child may use a tight, fixed pencil grasp and use arm and shoulder movements in order to form the designs rather than more efficient movements of the wrist and hand. The therapist may observe associated movements, such as overflow in the other hand or mouth and tongue movements. These unconscious movements may indicate that pencil-and-paper tasks are difficult for the child and require intense concentration. Extreme postural shifts made during the drawings may indicate an inability to cross the vertical midline of the body. Consequently, this child may be using increased effort to accomplish age-appropriate work. The therapist may note the child's approach to each drawing, observing whether the child uses several short lines to complete a design rather than longer, more efficient patterns.

Sensory Integration and Praxis Tests (SIPT)

The *Sensory Integration and Praxis Tests* (SIPT) (Ayres 1989) is a diagnostic battery designed to tease out the individual cluster of deficits which may contribute to a child's poor performance. Looking for clusters of problem performance areas makes it easier to analyze the child's overall performance. Looking for related problems is the first step toward successful remediation.

The SIPT is designed to be administered by an occupational or physical therapist with specialized training in sensory integration theory, test administration, and interpretation. Although the certification process is expensive and time-consuming, the information gained by the SIPT can be a valuable diagnostic tool. By determining the patterns of a child's poor performance, the therapist is able to establish an appropriate treatment plan.

This text is not designed to provide detailed information about the SIPT; specific manuals and training classes are designed to do that. Listed below are some of the subtests of this detailed battery. Brief descriptions are included to give the reader ideas about the types of information that may be obtained from this valuable tool.

- The Space Visualization and Figure-Ground subtests help sort out visual-spatial awareness difficulties.

- Design Copying and Motor Accuracy subtests require a motor response to visual stimuli. Comparisons may be drawn between a child's performance of these subtests to determine whether the difficulties are more related to visual perception or motor control.

- The Kinesthesia and Tactile subtests give the examiner information about the child's somatosensory or touch processing by assessing kinesthesia (sense of movement), tactile discrimination, and praxis (motor planning).

- Other subtests are indicators of vestibular processing and of the child's abilities in bilateral integration and sequencing.

Many school-based therapists are certified in the administration and interpretation of the SIPT. Those who are not may be able to contract with a private therapist to administer the SIPT. The SIPT examiner can aid the school-based therapist in establishing treatment guidelines that may be carried out or supplemented by the school.

In the absence of a standardized test like the SIPT for assessing motor-planning skills, the therapist may supplement traditional standardized evaluations, such as the Bruininks-Oseretsky *Test of Motor Proficiency* (Bruininks 1978) with clinical observation of the child's performance to better understand the child's motor-planning abilities. The *Miller Assessment for Preschoolers* (Miller 1988), DeGangi-Berk *Test of Sensory Integration* (1983), and the Peabody Assessment for Preschoolers in the *Peabody Developmental Motor Scales and Activity Cards* (Folio and Fewell 1983) also are excellent tests to obtain standardized data with supplemental clinical observations.

A major focus of this chapter is to review information already in use by skilled clinicians. By using familiar tools in conjunction with keen clinical observation skills, more information can be obtained about each child evaluated. Comparing and contrasting different test results will provide more information about the child's strengths and weaknesses. After the child's abilities and disabilities are clearly defined and understood, successful treatment planning and implementation can begin.

Bruininks-Oseretsky *Test of Motor Proficiency*

The following is a detailed description of the use of the Bruininks battery as a diagnostic tool to gather additional information about a child's motor planning, verbal comprehension, tactile sensitivity and sequencing. The Bruininks-Oseretsky *Test of Motor Proficiency* (Bruininks 1978) is a comprehensive battery including areas of fine motor and gross motor skill development. It is standardized for use with children between the ages of 4 and 15. Clinicians give the test in its standardized form and can supplement their findings through keen clinical observations.

The Bruininks manual directs the examiner to use the standardized instructions first; and then, if necessary, to assist the child by other means to perform each item. The type of assistance a child needs will provide insight into how the child will perform in a classroom situation. Children experiencing difficulties with verbal interpretation may not linguistically comprehend how to perform the task correctly. A child with difficulties performing the motor act may appear clumsy and uncoordinated. A child with sequencing difficulties may perform the task correctly, but use unnecessary steps or illogical sequencing to complete the job. Noting the child's performance style will provide invaluable clues to discovering the weak areas and, in turn, implementing a plan to help each child perform most effectively.

As the subtests of the Bruininks are reviewed, ideas for observing motor planning, verbal comprehension, tactile sensitivity, and sequencing are discussed. These four specific components are listed separately in this analysis of the Bruininks-Oseretsky test. These questions facilitate the reader's ability to analyze *what* is occurring during the performance of each item, to be able to look at *how* the task is performed and *why* a task was performed poorly. This information provides valuable insights into a child's ability to learn or to respond to new situations. One must look for *patterns* of performance among tests. For example, does the child:

- Consistently perform in a sloppy manner on fine and gross motor items (suggesting poor muscular control)?

- Need repeated visual demonstrations to complete the task (suggesting a poor ability to comprehend verbal instruction)?

- React negatively to touch (suggesting an overresponsive touch system; that is, tactual defensiveness)?

- Seem unable to perform the task in a logical or sequential fashion (suggesting motor-planning difficulties)?

Many items on the Bruininks battery require performance of tasks that have not been taught, learned, or practiced. These unique items are useful in assessing how the child responds to new, unfamiliar tasks. Take special note of the child's responses to those items in the testing; it may parallel how the child confronts new tasks presented in the classroom. It may be helpful to review the material presented in chapters 2 and 3; the terminology discussed in relation to the sensory integration systems and motor planning is incorporated in the following discussion.

The eight subtests of the Bruininks-Oseretsky *Test of Motor Proficiency* are discussed below. Recent research (Wilson 1995) suggests that the Running Speed and Agility, Balance, Visual-Motor Control, and Upper-Limb Speed and Dexterity subtests are likely to provide the greatest degree of discrimination between children with and without motor problems. However, all subtests are discussed in this chapter because of their unique skill requirements as pertaining to new motor-planning situations. Ideas for increasing observation skills are shared. Brief case studies are described to emphasize the importance of the additional observation. The children in the case studies were tested with the SIPT and Bruininks-Oseretsky. Their "occupational therapy diagnosis" was made after in-depth examination of both tests.

Running Speed and Agility Subtest

This subtest requires the child to run, retrieve an object, and return. The score is obtained by timing the running. The time score can be translated to an age equivalency. If a delayed score is noted, the examiner can begin to speculate about the reason for the delay. Was the child's difficulty related to poor interpretation of the verbal instructions, or poor motor execution of the task, or poor sequencing?

Clinical Considerations for Running Speed and Agility

Verbal interpretation
- Observe the child's posture as the task begins. Did the body "set" itself for the verbally explained task?

Motor performance (motor execution of the task)
- As the child ran, was there a reciprocal arm swing?

- As the child bent to pick up the vertically positioned block, were the movements executed smoothly, or were awkward movements observed?

The observation of a lack of postural setting to begin the task may suggest poor verbal comprehension or poor body positioning. Falling when retrieving the block may suggest poor motor planning or balance. Conversely, if the child executes the task smoothly without awkward movements, motor planning of these gross motor tasks may not be an issue and the child may just be a slow runner. Comparing and contrasting other subtests will result in similar performance areas to analyze.

Case Studies

Charles had been receiving occupational therapy and his test scores had improved to the point that discharge was considered. He performed the Running Speed and Agility Subtest in an average time for his age. However, his gait appeared awkward. He ran with a wide base and nearly lost his balance as he bent to retrieve the block. Despite an acceptable score, clinical observations substantiated the need to continue therapy to address the remaining motor-planning difficulties.

Travis, 6 years old, had been observed to run constantly. He frequently ran into objects and appeared to have poor protective responses. Although he had been observed to run "fast," he was unable to perform this subtest in an average amount of time for his age. He did not appear to have sufficient motor planning to perform a new task with control while running. A slight change in the task, which required him to bend over and retrieve a block, significantly lowered his skill performance.

Balance Subtest

Subitems include standing on one foot and standing on a balance beam with eyes open and eyes closed. Heel-to-toe walking is also required. The child also is asked to perform the unique task of stepping over a stick at knee height while walking the balance beam.

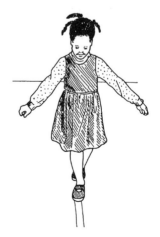

The item requiring the child to step over the stick will distinguish children who have been taught how to walk the balance beam from those who have good motor-planning and execution skills. Although the child's score is determined by the first two attempts, asking the child to continue to attempt the task allows the examiner to observe the child's motor learning.

Clinical Considerations for Balance

Verbal interpretation

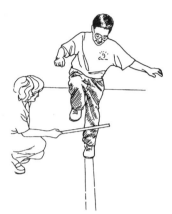

- Did the child perform the task appropriately after verbal directions, or was a physical demonstration required for the child to perform correctly?

Motor performance (motor execution of the task)

- Was the child's last attempt better than the first, or did repeated practice yield the same poor performance?

- Did the child appear to learn from earlier mistakes and make appropriate adjustments?

Sequencing of task

- When attempting to walk over the knee-height stick, was the child able to readjust stepping so that the feet were at the proper distance to step?

- Was the child able to perform the required steps slowly and smoothly?

Tactile sensitivity

- Did the child become ticklish when physical assistance was provided?

- Was the child startled when touched on the leg or foot without being aware that you were about to physically assist?

Some children, despite numerous attempts, cannot execute the task. Other children can perform only when walking fast. When they are required to perform the task slowly, performance decreases. Continued observation will help to clarify the reasons behind each child's failures. Poor balance may be the primary reason. In other cases, inefficient motor planning in this new situation may cause poor performance.

Case Studies

Although Justin was 12, he was not able to walk the balance beam for six consecutive steps. He practiced and was determined to succeed. His poor balance, in combination with his decreased body awareness and poor motor-planning abilities, made this task impossible.

Parents and teachers reported that Peter, 12 years old, had good motor skills. He had been honored with a few Physical Education awards and was becoming interested in competitive diving. However, his balance subtest score was low. He was unable to successfully step over the stick while walking the balance beam. When he was required to use particular skills in new situations, skill levels significantly decreased until he had sufficient time to practice. This scenario was also noted in other areas; he was resistive to learning new games and had extremely slow handwriting. When analyzing these instances with parents and teachers, the therapist pointed out that although the skills were good, Peter appeared to need extra time to practice and "think through" new situations.

Bilateral Coordination Subtest

In this subtest, the examiner verbally describes and visually demonstrates the test items. Although this reduces the examiner's ability to note problems with auditory interpretations, the uniqueness of the test components permits countless opportunities for noting execution and sequencing of the motor tasks. A child with poor bilateral integration will perform poorly on this task. However, a child with good bilateral integration but poor motor execution skills also may perform poorly. Due to the complexity of these subitems, it is difficult to determine whether the motor execution problems are due to poor bilateral integration, sequencing, or motor execution of the task.

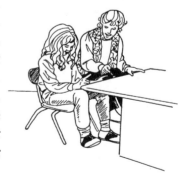

Observing the child throughout the complete battery will assist in determining the child's area of weakness. Clinical experience has suggested that children with adequate bilateral integration skills who have difficulty with motor planning may appear disappointed or frustrated. Children with poor bilateral integration make little attempt to perform the tasks demonstrated. They seem to sense that the tasks are too involved for their skill level.

Case Studies

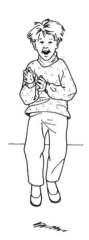

Jennifer was a second grader who appeared to be struggling in all areas of school. Her teachers described her as slow and lethargic. Her speech was labored and her tongue moved awkwardly. Her handwriting was large and jerky. As she performed jumping jacks, her arms and legs did not move smoothly. She appeared to be stuck to the floor when trying to jump. Complete evaluation suggested poor bilateral integration as well as poor motor planning and gravitational insecurity. Poor motor skills in addition to bilateral integration made learning and performance very difficult for this young girl.

Martha was determined to get a fast score on the subitem of drawing lines and crosses simultaneously. She talked herself through each motion ("Both hands together, right hand cross; both hands together, right hand cross"). Her subtest score was in a low-average range. However, clinically it was necessary to explain that she achieved this score by going to extraordinary means. This was how she accomplished her work in school. Despite her poor motor-planning skills, her intelligence was sufficient to allow her to talk herself through difficult motor situations. Although she was "making it in school," she came home exhausted and frustrated.

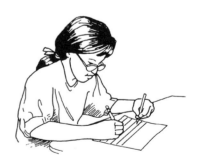

Strength Subtest

The tasks included in the strength subtest are familiar to many children. However, they have components which make them unique motor-planning tests. The standing broad jump uses a mat to define the child's spatial boundaries. The sit-ups are similar to half-sit-ups with a varied arm position. The knee push-ups are required for all children under age 8. The examiner may choose to administer this item to older boys as a clinical observation (not included in the scoring).

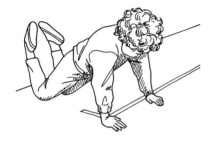

Although children may have performed sit-ups and push-ups, the Bruininks-Oseretsky test slightly changes the physical components to present good opportunities for the clinician to observe motor planning.

Clinical Considerations for Strength

Motor performance (motor execution of the task)

- Are the child's jumps awkward?

- Does the child consistently land unbalanced?

- Can the child perform the arm "pump" motions in a manner that facilitates the broad jump?

- How much physical assistance is required to assume the positions for the sit-ups or push-ups?

- How easily can the child maneuver into position going from sit-ups to push-ups?

Sequencing of task

- Children with poor sequencing may have an arrhythmic "pump." Did the child jump at the correct position of the arm "pump" sequence?

- Is the child able to readapt to the changes in the arm position on the sit-ups without needing verbal reminders?

Tactile sensitivity

- Does the child tolerate physical assistance from the examiner to assume the correct position?

- Does the child respond negatively to physical prompting?

A deficit score in the Strength Subtest may suggest overall weakness, or it may be an indication of the child's flexor or extensor muscle functions. Inability to perform sit-ups may be due to poor integration of the tonic labyrinthine reflex (which allows a child to move against the pull of gravity) or poor flexor tone. Inability to assume the push-up position may be due to weak back and neck extensor muscles.

Case Studies

Johnny, 6 years old, was unable to get his feet off the floor for the standing broad jump. His parents reported he had not been observed to jump. He was reluctant to climb stairs and did not climb on playground equipment. Although his final Strength Subtest score was in a low-average range, further testing revealed severe discomfort in response to movement against gravity, termed *gravitational insecurity.*

Sandra appeared to be a strong girl with good muscle tone. However, she was unable to perform neck flexion to initiate a sit-up. Further testing suggested a poorly integrated tonic labyrinthine reflex in the supine position.

Upper-Limb Coordination Subtest

The testing items included on this subtest are primarily ball catching and tossing.

Other items assess finger coordination. Many of these items are familiar to children, so limited information about verbal comprehension can be obtained. Clinically, this subtest seems to be the most frustrating for the child with poor motor execution skills.

Clinical Considerations for Upper-Limb Coordination

Motor performance (motor execution of the task)

- Was the child able to position the body properly in order to catch the ball? Although the examiner throws the ball to the child from a distance of 10 feet, the child with poor motor execution may move inappropriately during the attempt to catch the ball.

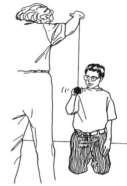

- If the child goes to retrieve the ball, observe maneuverability in the room and around obstacles.

- Does continued practice for tapping the swinging ball produce improved results, or does practice only prove to be more frustrating?

Sequencing of task

- While attempting to touch fingertip to nose, does the child try to use alternate hands or use random motions?

- Did the child perform the finger pivoting in a natural sequence, or were fingers moved randomly?

Tactile sensitivity

- How does the child respond if the ball inadvertently hits the child's body?

- Is the child resistive to the examiner physically assisting to demonstrate an item?

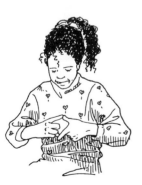

- Ask the child if it is easier to perform nose- and finger-touching with eyes open or eyes closed.

- Does the child appear to have good kinesthesia to touch fingertip to nose in a smooth and precise manner?

Case Studies

Lauren, a developmentally delayed 5-year-old, appeared to have no idea what to do with her hands as the ball approached her. Comprehensive testing suggested that she had poor sensory feedback, poor motor planning, and poor eye-hand coordination. She also had no idea about how to use her hands to interact with new toys or climb on equipment.

Karl was unable to catch the ball. He threw it to the examiner hard and with poor control. After many throws, his accuracy and control showed no improvement. SIPT testing revealed a poor kinesthesia subtest performance. Other somatosensory tests also were performed poorly. Karl's inability to sense his arm position caused a wide variety in his attempts to throw the ball.

Response Speed Subtest

This subtest may be the most unique of all the Bruininks-Oseretsky items. Verbal and visual instructions are given. This subtest requires the child to stop a vertically moving stick with an isolated thumb motion. It provides a wonderful opportunity to observe the child performing a new motor task for the first time.

Motor performance (execution) difficulties may be observed in a child who is unable to perform the required thumb retraction. Some younger children are unable to perform this retraction, while older children may

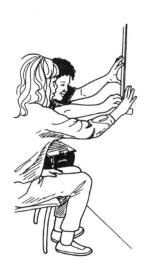

maneuver the thumb awkwardly. Other children may have difficulty assuming or maintaining their body and hand positions. Continued practice may improve their scores. Record the test performance as required. The examiner may choose to continue the "game" to observe the child's motor learning skills.

Children with sequencing difficulties may consistently be "off" in their timing. These children may not wish to continue to practice because they seem to sense it is too difficult for them.

Interestingly, comparison and contrast data discussed in the literature accompanying the Bruininks-Oseretsky test state that there was no significant difference between the mean scores of normal subjects and learning disabled subjects on this subtest (Bruininks 1978, 34).

Ask how frequently the child plays video games. The child's score on this subtest may be artificially enhanced by video game practice.

Many parents ask, "Should I buy a video game set for my child to improve fine motor skills?" We feel strongly that although playing video games may increase finger dexterity, motor skills are improved most effectively by an overall body coordination program, including sensory integration techniques when appropriate.

Case Study

Damon tried repeatedly to stop the stick with his thumb. He firmly stated to the examiner, "Can't you see my hands aren't good enough to do this?" Further testing showed decreased finger dexterity as well as poor motor planning in gross motor and fine motor areas.

Visual-Motor Control Subtest

This subtest is primarily a pencil-and-paper test. It is untimed (although the examiner may wish to time the items to compare during later reevaluation). One item requires the child to cut out a circle accurately. Other items call for the child to copy geometric designs. A therapist experienced in watching children draw will gain valuable information by noting directionality, crossing the midline, and sequencing.

Clinical Considerations for Visual-Motor Control

Motor performance (motor execution of the task)

- Is the handwriting shaky or wavy?
- Observe the pencil grasp. Is it awkward? Is it too tight?
- Does the pencil grasp change during the drawing process?
- Does the child attempt to reorient the paper to avoid crossing the midline?
- Does the child reorient body position to avoid crossing the midline?

Sequencing of task

- Although instructed where to begin, does the child start in a different location?
- Do the pencil drawings overlap unnecessarily? This may indicate poor sequencing and inefficient strokes.
- Is the picture drawn in an unusual sequence?

Case Studies

Letricia was referred for evaluation by an occupational therapist after her tutor of three years became concerned about her slowness in completing written work. In addition to the SIPT, selected subtests of the Bruininks were administered. Although she was actually 8 years old, her score on Running Speed and Agility fell in the 4-year-old range. Her Visual-Motor Control score fell in the 7-year-old range. Clinical observation of her approach to the drawings on the Visual-Motor Control Subtest showed that she did not draw in a left-right progression. The evaluating therapist had timed her performance on the visual-motor items. This information helped the teachers, tutor, and parents decide to temporarily reduce the amount of written work they required of Letricia. As therapy progressed, the time required for her to write decreased, while the neatness and accuracy of her work increased.

Calvin was participating in the regular third grade in his public school. He had been accepted into and was participating in the gifted and talented program. However, his written work was very poor. His mother reported that he had been coming home from school in tears because he hated to write. His teachers felt he was being lazy by not writing more neatly ("After all, he's a bright boy").

Complete testing using the Bruininks-Oseretsky (to give the public school age-equivalency performances) and the SIPT (to provide additional diagnostic and treatment information) produced interesting results. Calvin's gross motor scores on the Bruininks were in the average range. His fine motor scores were in the 5- to 6-year-old range, suggesting a delay of three to four years. His SIPT results suggested poor vestibular processing. Decreased vestibular processing seemed to have negatively affected his cerebral hemispheres with respect to lateralizing fine motor skills. Although he was primarily performing fine motor work as a right-handed child, his left hand could perform each task equally well. He did not have a dominant hand.

Treatment planning included primarily vestibular activities during his private occupational therapy sessions. His occupational therapist in the public school reviewed the test results with teachers. Handwriting requirements were decreased. As his handwriting required less effort and became neater, the teacher's expectations were gradually increased.

Upper-Limb Speed and Dexterity Subtest

These test items allow the therapist to observe the child's fine motor manipulative abilities and assign a time factor to the performance. Verbal instructions allow the therapist to obtain more information about the child's auditory abilities. The complexity of the items permits wonderful opportunities to observe the child's organizational and sequencing skills.

Clinical Considerations for Upper-Limb Speed and Dexterity

Motor performance (motor execution of task)

- Does the child's approach appear clumsy? (For example, pennies missing the box when attempting to toss pennies, inability to keep the sorted cards in stacks, dropping the beads during attempts to string them, or knocking out the pegs in the pegboard)

- Are the pencil marks messy?

Sequencing of task

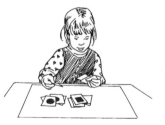

- Does the child seem to put extra effort into performing these tasks?

- Are the items picked up randomly?

- Does the child have an established sequence to string beads, or are the hands switched frequently?

- Are the pegs moved in an apparent sequence, or are they moved randomly?

- Although the time score may be within acceptable levels, did the child require extra effort to accomplish the tasks?

Verbal interpretations

- Was the child able to follow your verbal directions, or were visual cues necessary to obtain acceptable performance?

Case Study

Andy was 12 when he was evaluated, using the SIPT, Bruininks-Oseretsky, and Beery-Buktenica *Test of Visual-Motor Integration*. Although Andy's occupational therapy testing in his local public school did not qualify him for services, his parents elected to have him attend private occupational therapy. Consequently, despite his fine and gross motor delays, accommodations to his junior high environment were going to be minimum. Like many other children, his IQ tested high and academically Andy was not having difficulty "keeping up." However, he was not able to write neatly or as quickly as his peers, he was having difficulty fingering his trumpet, and his delayed gross motor skills were beginning to embarrass him in Physical Education. He came home from school physically exhausted and frustrated. The private occupational therapist, at the parents' request, was able to review Andy's testing with his school counselor. Although she was skeptical of these "outside" assessments, the similarity of the *Wechsler Intelligence Scale for Children—Revised*, Coding subtest (Wechsler 1974), to an item in the Upper-Limb Speed and Dexterity subtest seemed to increase her respect for the other data. Andy's teachers decreased the amount of written work required of him. Typing skills were planned in his curriculum ahead of his peers. The counselor agreed to share the summary of the occupational therapy results with Andy's teachers, and to work to minimize damage to Andy's self-esteem. Andy wanted to continue to play the trumpet, but elected to play with the concert band rather than to attempt the marching band.

It is important to look for patterns throughout the entire battery rather than observe one subtest and assume that the child's difficulties are due to one isolated area of motor planning. By observing how the child performs the varied tasks of this battery, you can provide a wealth of information to the parents and teachers about how the child is functioning.

Miller Assessment for Preschoolers

Although the *Miller Assessment for Preschoolers* (Miller 1988) requires additional training to administer, it seems to be more accessible than the SIPT. It is an invaluable resource in working with children not clearly identified as having a learning, motor, or verbal difficulty. The Miller test is standardized to administer to children between the ages of 2 years 9 months to 5 years 8 months.

Research has substantiated the predictive validity of this assessment (Miller, Cohn, and Lemerand 1988). Having this resource available may be helpful in obtaining services for at-risk children.

As with the Bruininks-Oseretsky test, the Miller should be performed in standardized form. Additional observations can be used to look for patterns of strengths and weaknesses in each child's performance. Some of the most useful items for looking at patterns of motor planning and sequencing are discussed below.

1. **Tower**—The child is directed to stack 1-inch cubes.

   The child's approach to building the tower is helpful in assessing the child's sequencing skills. Ask the child to assist in putting the blocks back into the box, and observe how organized and sequenced that task is performed. Is the child able to cross midline?

5. **Stereognosis**—The child is asked to identify familiar items without seeing them.

   Observe how well the child is able to manipulate the items. As the child is handed the items without being able to see them, are tactile defensive responses noted?

6. **Finger Localization**—The child is asked to point to a finger touched by the examiner.

   Does the child respond to the examiner's touch in a defensive manner? Does the child appear to have sufficient kinesthesia to point to the correct finger?

8. **Puzzle**—The child is asked to assemble a two- or three-part puzzle.

   How does the child manipulate the puzzle pieces? Does the child learn from errors and change the motor plan, or are the same errors repeated?

10. **Draw a Person**—The child is given a sheet of paper and crayons and asked to "draw a person."

    How well does the child respond to your verbal directions? Does the child use the space on the paper appropriately?

11. **Cage**—The child is asked to draw a series of vertical lines.

    Observe the pencil grasp. Does it change frequently? How is the child controlling the pencil?

12. **Vertical Writing**—The child is asked to draw a series of short lines from the top of the page to the bottom.

    This item is performed with vision occluded. Does the child have a fear of attempting the task because of a poor sense of kinesthesia?

14. **Rhomberg**—The child is asked to stand with feet together in "heel-to-toe" position.

    This test item also is performed with vision occluded. Can the child balance while standing on two feet with vision occluded? Is the child fearful of attempting the task? Is there a correlation to other balance items?

15. **Stepping**—The child is asked to march in place.

    Can the child verbally comprehend the task? Does a lack of proprioception or kinesthesia prevent the child from attempting this item?

17. **Supine flexion**—The child is placed in a back-lying position and asked to curl up knees, hips, and neck.

    Does the child allow the examiner to physically assist with the position? How well can the child maneuver in and out of the position?

18. **Kneel to Stand**—The child is asked to rise to standing from a kneeling position.

    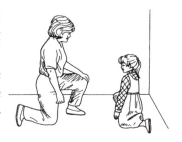

    As the child attempts this task, observe for extra postural adjustments. Was the child able to comprehend the verbal directions?

19. **Imitation of Postures**—The child is asked to assume body positions modeled by the examiner.

How quickly is the child able to assume the new body postures? Does the child appear to be "thinking through" the motions, or can the movements occur almost spontaneously?

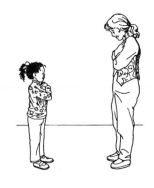

22. **Maze**—The child is asked to solve a simple two- or three-dimensional maze by tilting or turning it.

    Do subsequent attempts at the maze show that the child has made motor adaptations to the task? Does the child repeat the same errors?

24. **Following Directions**—The child is asked to respond to directions given by the examiner.

    This subtest provides a clear indication of verbal abilities to perform new motor planning. How easily can the child manipulate the items?

25. **Articulation**—The child is asked to repeat a series of words.

    Oral motor skills and tongue motor planning are easily observed on this subtest. Frequently children with slower gross and fine motor planning will also display slow oral-motor articulation.

Case Study

Ronald displayed left hemiparesis at birth due to a cerebral cyst. He received therapy primarily for increasing left-hand use, maintaining the passive range of motion and increasing his active range of motion. As he was about to begin preschool, a developmental assessment was requested. At 3 years, 10 months, his performance was in average ranges with the exception of poor supine flexion, kneel to stand, and finger identification. He was not able to perform the task with his eyes closed on any of the items requesting vision occluded.

After this assessment, a pattern of questionable vestibular processing was suspected. (The difficulties with supine flexion, balance, and inability to balance without vision are all vestibular related functions.) His original therapy plan was modified to include activities to improve vestibular processing. Including more sensorimotor activities in his original therapy plan helped to improve his overall skills required to succeed in preschool.

DeGangi-Berk *Test of Sensory Integration*

The DeGangi-Berk *Test of Sensory Integration* (1983) is standardized for children ages 3 to 5. It is designed to assess postural control, bilateral motor integration, and reflex integration in preschool children. It was constructed as a criterion-referenced test to be administered with children with delays in sensory, motor, and perceptual skills or to children suspected of having learning problems.

Monkey Task—The child is asked to hang horizontally from a long dowel rod by holding on with hands and crossing legs.

This task assesses the ability to assume and maintain a flexed posture against the pull of gravity.

Side-Sit Co-contraction—The child is asked to hold a side-sitting position while the examiner pushes in the opposite direction.

This task assesses how the muscle groups of the arms and trunk work together.

Rolling-Pin Activity—The child is asked to hold a rolling pin with both hands and hit a suspended ball.

This task assesses a child's ability to use both hands together, rotate the trunk, and cross the body's midline.

Prone on Elbows—The child is asked to lie face down supported on the elbows facing a picture.

This task assesses the ability to maintain neck position against the pull of gravity.

Wheelbarrow Walk—The child is asked to walk on hands while the examiner supports the feet.

This task assesses stability of the neck, trunk, and upper extremity extensors.

Airplane—The therapist supports the child in a face-down position and asks the child to extend the arms and "fly."

This task assesses the ability to hold an extension posture against the pull of gravity.

Jump and Turn—The child is asked to jump up and complete a 180-degree turn.

This activity assesses bilateral motor coordination of the lower extremities and trunk rotation.

Scooterboard Co-contraction—The child is asked to sit cross-legged on a scooterboard and move the board by pushing against the examiner's hands.

This task assesses balance between muscle groups of the shoulders and arms.

Asymmetrical Tonic Neck Reflex Integration—The child is asked to assume a hands-and-knees position while the examiner turns the child's head.

The examiner observes for bending of the elbow of the opposite arm.

Symmetrical Tonic Neck Reflex Integration—The child is asked to assume a hands-and-knees position while the examiner moves the child's head up and down.

The examiner observes for isolated head and trunk movement.

Diadokokinesia—The child is asked to perform rapidly alternating hand movements.

This task assesses the ability to rotate the forearms in a smooth and coordinated manner.

Drumming—The child is asked to perform rhythmic alternating hand movements.

This task assesses the ability to use the two sides of the body in a smooth and coordinated manner.

Upper-Extremity Control—The child is asked to trace a star design.

This task assesses motor speed, the ability to isolate trunk and arm movements, and crossing midline functions.

Peabody Developmental Motor Scales

This battery (Folio and Fewell 1983) contains gross motor and fine motor scales for children from birth to 6 years. The test items vary with developmental age. The test manual contains instructions for administration, including level, item, child's position, directions, and criteria. The Peabody may be used in conjunction with the Miller or DeGangi-Berk tests to measure change over time. The examiner may make important clinical observations as to the quality of a child's movements on items such as grasping, placing pegs, and removing socks. Novel items such as building a bridge with 1-inch cubes may be used as an indicator of praxis or motor-planning abilities.

Case Study

Anthony was referred for occupational therapy evaluation at 2½ years due to suspected delays in developmental milestones secondary to a congenital heart defect. His initial evaluation consisted of the *Miller Assessment for Preschoolers*. His scores fell primarily within the at-risk range with particularly low scores on the Foundations and Coordination indices. Clinical observations suggested tactual defensiveness and motor-planning deficits. After approximately six months of treatment, the *Peabody Developmental Motor Scales* were administered, which showed mild delays in both gross motor and fine motor skills. Portions of the DeGangi-Berk were administered to assess sensory integration.

At 3 years, in addition to his therapy program, Anthony was enrolled in an early childhood program in his public school. This program provided speech therapy, adaptive P.E., and early learning readiness. He continued to receive occupational therapy on a private basis until age 4, at which time his scores fell within normal limits in all areas assessed. At age 5, he was screened for public kindergarten and found to be on-level in his physical and academic readiness for kindergarten. He has continued to attend public school without further intervention.

Clinical Observations Frequently Associated with Sensory Integration Testing

A Guide to Testing Clinical Observations in Kindergartners (Dunn 1981) is an excellent reference for correct administration of the following items.

Co-contraction—The child is asked to maintain body position while the examiner gently pushes in different directions.

This test helps to analyze the child's ability to use the flexor and extensor muscle groups in a reciprocal balance. For example, to successfully control the arm for writing, the muscles co-contract to create a balance for motor control.

Supine Flexion—The child is asked to assume a back-lying position and curl up at knees, hips, and neck.

This tonic muscle position assesses primitive reflex integration which allows movement against the pull of gravity as well as the body's flexor muscle tone.

Prone Extension—The child is asked to lift head, arms, and legs off the floor while lying on the stomach.

This tonic muscle position assesses primitive reflex integration which allows movement against the pull of gravity as well as the body's extensor muscle tone. This muscle group works continuously to keep the body upright against gravity. A child with poor extensor tone will most likely need to hold up the head with one hand because the neck extensor fatigues quickly.

Diadokokinesia—The child is asked to perform rapidly alternating arm and hand movements.

This rapid repetitive motion provides much information about each child's ability to learn a new motor task, perform a quick motion, and use both sides of the body simultaneously in a smooth and coordinated pattern.

Postural Security—The child is asked to sit atop a large therapy ball moved gently by the examiner.

Children normally feel comfortable moving freely in their environment, swinging, jumping, rolling, and reclining. When a child feels fearful, insecure, anxious, or uncomfortable about moving, the child is called *posturally insecure* or *gravitationally insecure*. This is directly correlated to the vestibular system function.

Protective Extension—The child is asked to lie face down on a large therapy ball which the examiner moves forward quickly.

When a person falls, usually the hands come out automatically to protect the body and face. When this occurs spontaneously, children are believed to have sufficient protective extension. However, when this response does not occur subconsciously and spontaneously, an increased rate of injury often results. This is directly related to the vestibular system function.

CHAPTER 5

Treatment Ideas

A complete evaluation is the first step of any treatment program. A child experiencing learning and/or attention problems may require evaluations by numerous professionals (medical, educational, psychosocial) in order to gather a complete "picture" of the situation. Next, this team of professionals, together with the parents, must establish a plan focusing on the total child's needs. The more information available about how the child "works," the easier it will be to understand the idiosyncrasies of the child's behavior, as well as strengths and weaknesses in learning abilities.

The treatment ideas discussed in this chapter are primarily sensorimotor related. These sensorimotor activities are reviewed for the classroom, clinic, and home settings.

Treatment for a child with learning disability may occur in many settings. A child may be seen primarily by the school-based occupational therapist or by a therapist in a private clinic. Many therapists provide a home program to be carried out by the parents to supplement and support the child's treatment plan. In this chapter we offer a sampler of treatment ideas which may be carried out as a part of a formal therapy session or in a less formal setting such as the home or playground.

The term *treatment ideas* is a large concept to address. For the purposes of this manual, we will present a variety of treatment activities that can be used in a variety of settings. Treatment, from our perspective, should be suited to fit the individual child's need to "make things go better." Treatment of a child with learning disability may be as simple as understanding why a child may react to a new situation, or as complex as interventions that involve medication, counseling, and therapy.

Chapter 5 is divided into three idea areas: Classroom Games, Home Strategies, and Therapeutic Activities. Many of the activities can be modified to be used in other situations. These activities are not cookbook ideas to try on each child; rather, they are listed as references to stimulate the therapist, parent, or teacher to use the idea and expand it appropriately for the individual child.

All of these treatment ideas require the therapist, parent, or teacher to look at the whole child and briefly assess the child and situation on that day. What may be calming to a child one day may be overstimulating the next. A review of chapter 2, Sensory Systems, may be helpful as we discuss how the different sensory systems affect children. The tactile system and its responses to light and firm touch will create a variety of responses from a child. How well a child is able to feel how an arm or leg has moved and how the body is positioned (kinesthesia and proprioception) will provide information to the teacher, parent, or therapist about how that child will respond to an activity. The balance and motion-detection areas in the ear (vestibular system) have direct connections to areas of the body affecting digestion and muscle tone as well as emotion. If each child is not being observed and understood individually, the child may not be receiving appropriate treatment. Treatment performed to address an identified problem may produce positive or negative effects in other areas. The therapist, parent, and teacher must be trained to observe the whole child!

For the remainder of this chapter, the term *therapist* will be used to mean the person guiding the therapeutic activity. That "therapist" may be the occupational or physical therapist, speech-language pathologist, parent, or teacher. Observing the whole child requires the therapist to think of all the sensory systems together. Besides observing how the child is responding to a specific touch or movement activity, the therapist must be aware of the environment and the child's mood. This is no easy task! However, it is important to "tune in" to the child and become aware of the whole world affecting school performance. A complete evaluation by an appropriately trained therapist will give the "treating therapist" knowledge as to whether the child tends to be overresponsive to touch (tactually defensive) or is more unaware of touch. This evaluation also should provide the treating therapist vital information about how the child is able to sense body position and how that child perceives and accommodates to space in the environment (spatial awareness). Here are a few questions to help the therapist assess those less-clearly defined areas such as environment and mood.

Does the child:

- Have a calm, relaxing morning before coming to school?

- Attend morning care before coming to school?

- Ride the bus? If so, how stimulating is the ride?

- Have comfortable clothes? (This is most important for the child who is oversensitive to touch.)

- Feel safe and secure in the learning environment?

- Feel physically well and healthy?

There may be no better way to explain how to "put all the sensory systems together" than to use an analogy. Imagine yourself in your normal routine day. Think of all the things you are able to accomplish and all of the interruptions you are able to accommodate. On a normal day you can be creative and innovative and can think quickly.

Now recall a day when you were not feeling up to par. Perhaps you were coming down with the flu. Were you able to accomplish your normal tasks? Did you become easily irritated by interruptions? Did you attempt your work only to find unsatisfactory results? Perhaps to feel better you treated yourself to a cup of hot tea in a quiet room beneath a comforter. One seemingly small difference in the routine caused a major change in your abilities and needs for a day.

Although this is a simplistic example, our children with learning and attention problems are generally working so hard to perform their best each day that one seemingly minor change to the routine (the wrong shirt, a substitute teacher, Mother out of town, a torn paper) may make a completely different need to be addressed by the treatment regime. Sometimes it becomes necessary to substitute an alternate activity which is more appropriate than the one that had been planned.

Our nervous system functions in a balance. When all is equal and functioning smoothly, we function at our optimum state.

Optimum Functioning Day

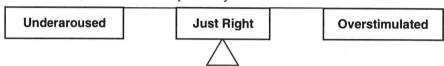

Normal, average muscle tone
Refreshed, ready to perform appearance
Appropriate tone and speed to speech
Interacting appropriately with others
Normal heart rate
Not too calm, not too excited,
just ready to learn

Underaroused	Just Right	Overstimulated

In the example, the flu caused a disequilibrium in the optimum state. Because the equilibrium was interrupted, the ability to think creatively, tune out distractions, have an appropriate mood, and function normally was compromised. The same is true for a child who has a nervous system in disequilibrium. A child who is bored, almost asleep, fatigued, depressed, or withdrawn may be termed *underaroused*. If bouncing off the walls, irritable, showing increased muscle tone and tension, "wired," or jumpy, the child may be termed *overstimulated*. In either case, the child will not be functioning at an optimum level for the nervous system to produce appropriate tasks required for school or home.

Underaroused State

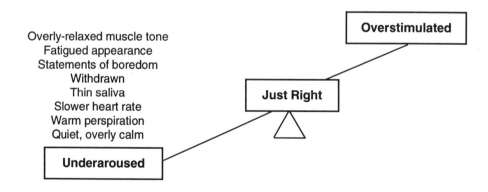

Overly-relaxed muscle tone
Fatigued appearance
Statements of boredom
Withdrawn
Thin saliva
Slower heart rate
Warm perspiration
Quiet, overly calm

Overstimulated State

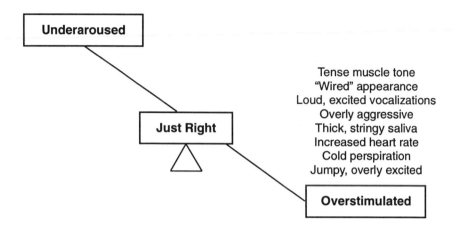

Tense muscle tone
"Wired" appearance
Loud, excited vocalizations
Overly aggressive
Thick, stringy saliva
Increased heart rate
Cold perspiration
Jumpy, overly excited

The daily treatment assessment is centered around this equilibrium in the nervous system. When the therapist plays a key role in helping each child reach the appropriate equilibrium for learning, treatment ideas can be incorporated into each child's needs. By noting a tilt in the equilibrium in one direction, the therapist can counterbalance with appropriate activities that promote the other end of the continuum. Two case studies will clarify this need to evaluate each child each day to help obtain the optimum balance.

Ryan, age 8, was diagnosed at 2 years old with mild cerebral palsy. He had received extensive physical therapy utilizing Neurodevelopmental Treatment (NDT) techniques. Ryan had attended kindergarten at a private school, but he came to public school for first grade. He was receiving consulting occupational therapy, direct physical therapy, and adaptive P.E. services. Ryan was integrated into the regular first grade classroom and was pulled from class for speech therapy twice weekly. He was able to walk independently, using a "scissor-type" gait at a slightly slower rate than his peers. Modifications were made for writing and other fine motor requirements. Ryan was socially well accepted and seemed to be fitting in well to his new situation. However, his teacher began to notice that he was coming to school agitated and seemed to be having more trouble sitting and attending to his school work. The occupational and physical therapist consultants were asked to evaluate the situation.

At the beginning part of each school day, Ryan's muscle tone was increased more than it had been at the beginning of the school year, he was drooling thick saliva, he spoke loudly, and was having difficulties attending to the teacher. Investigation revealed that Ryan's previous bus ride of 5 minutes had changed to a 20-minute bus ride. The stimulating atmosphere and jerky movements of the bus were increasing his muscle tone and excitement level. The situation was remedied by having his mother drive him to school. Ryan's muscle tone decreased to manageable levels and his attention level increased. However, he was disappointed that his mother no longer let him ride the bus. In this example, a simple analysis of Ryan's environment could explain his sudden change in readiness for learning.

Since she was 2 years old, Fran had been receiving occupational therapy addressing her sensory-integrative deficits. At age 3, speech therapy was initiated to address her language delays. Her sensory integration evaluation revealed developmental delays in all areas tested. Other developmental testing performed when she was 2 years old suggested her performance level in the 12-month range. Fran received speech therapy immediately after her twice-weekly occupational therapy sessions. When Fran arrived at her occupational therapy session, usually she was lethargic, relaxed, and uninterested in activity. In the initial minutes of her occupational therapy treatment, the therapist used activities that were designed to arouse and excite her lethargic nervous system.

One day, the speech therapist requested that Fran attend speech prior to occupational therapy because of a scheduling conflict. It quickly became apparent to the speech therapist that the activities performed in occupational therapy before speech therapy prepared Fran for a more productive speech therapy session. The speech therapist rearranged her schedule to continue seeing Fran after occupational therapy.

Looking at the seesaw of equilibrium in the nervous system can provide the therapy clues needed to begin treatment. For example, when the seesaw is tilted in the direction of an overaroused child, activities should be provided that promote the responses noted on the calming end of the seesaw.

When you see a child who appears to be:
    Loud
    "Bouncing off the walls"
    Easily irritated by noise
    Complaining of people touching him
    Anxious to hit something
    Unable to sit in the classroom seat

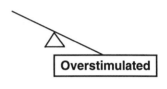

initiate activities designed to calm the nervous system, such as:
    Deep-touch pressure
    Dim lighting in the room
    Slow rocking (rocking chair in the classroom?)
    Quiet time in a secluded area of the classroom
    Carrying books for the teacher and other heavy work

However, if the seesaw is tilted in the opposite direction of underarousal and the child appears to be:
    Lethargic
    Bored
    Holding the head up with the arms
    Using slow, monotone speech
    Using a "closed," withdrawn posture

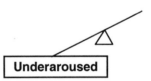

initiate activities that stimulate the nervous system to equalize, such as:
    Vigorous tactile rubbing
    Jumping
    Activities that involve bright lights and colors
    Bouncing on a trampoline or mat
    Lively music

By attempting to equalize the balance of the nervous system, the child should be more prepared to learn in school or perform appropriately at home.

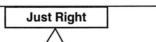

We hope these treatment ideas will encourage therapists, teachers, and parents to be creative when working or playing with their children who have special needs. By understanding the relationship between the arousal level of the nervous system, the environment, and the activity, we can help children to succeed.

Many of the games that follow have been created by the precious children who have taught us so much. Thanks to all of them.

Now enjoy the games!

Classroom Games

Feely Bag

This game requires a paper bag and a different small item for each member of the class. Items could include paper clips, a comb, a leaf, a penny, a crayon, and other items. One item is placed in each bag, and the bags are numbered. Each class member identifies the item in each bag by using the sense of touch, putting a hand inside the bag to feel the items without seeing them.

Implications: This activity helps to develop the child's sense of discriminatory touch.

Fun Day

One teacher frequently rewards her whole class by allowing each child to choose a sensorimotor activity after good behavior during the week. Some children put shaving cream on their desks and draw or practice making letters. Others choose modeling clay to make sculptures. Still others use small rocks to make letters and pictures.

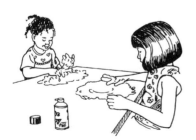

Implications: Each child chooses a tactile activity that is best suited to that child's needs. The tactually defensive child who resists unusual textures probably would not choose shaving cream, but perhaps might draw with rocks.

Cleaning up after Fun Day can be a tactile activity, too. Make hand brushes available for added touch input.

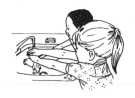

Jump-Rope Letters

Place a line of masking tape on the floor. Have each child use a jump rope to form a cursive letter, using the entire length of the rope. As skill levels increase, provide longer pieces of string, and have the children write words.

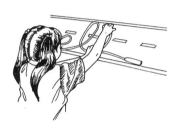

Implications: Motor planning and sequencing are practiced during this activity. Note how each child is able to sequence and plan how to use the correct amount of rope for each letter so that the entire letter can be formed or word can be spelled.

Clap-Snap

While waiting for an assembly to begin, a teacher involved three classrooms of first graders by playing a clap-snap game. The teacher clapped out a rhythm pattern, and the children repeated it. As the game progressed, the patterns became more complex. If someone was not able to keep up with the rest of the group, it seemed to go unnoticed because the group of children was intent on watching the next clap-snap pattern.

Implications: This is another game that gives the children an opportunity to practice sequencing as well as body coordination involving both sides of the body working together (bilateral integration).

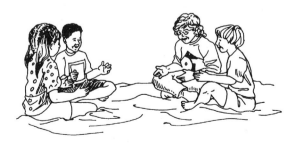

Reading Corner

Ideally, each classroom has a space for children to relax among pillows and read. In some classrooms where there have been a few overly aroused children, the teacher has acquired two dishwasher-sized boxes and filled them with pillows. When one of the six sides of the box is removed, there are many ways to turn the box to accommodate the needs of a variety of children. For the overly aroused child, getting completely inside the box in the dark quiet may assist in the calming. Other children may prefer to stretch out on the pillows and read with fewer visual and auditory distractions. Still others may just want to be out of sight of their peers and get underneath the pillows to calm themselves.

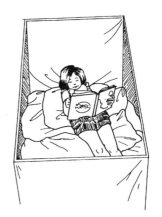

Implications: The box provides an opportunity for the overly aroused child to balance the nervous system equilibrium seesaw with some calming activities. Given the countless ways to use the box environment, many children can find a way to fix the box to help them calm down.

Home Strategies

When suggesting a home program, it is important to remember that the parent has more important roles to play with a child than therapist. After all, parenting is the hardest job of all, and no one else can fulfill that role. We believe that it may be more effective for the therapist to provide information to the parents rather than prescribe frequently ineffective home programs. We recommend the old Cub Scout adage, KISMIF (Keep It Simple, Make It Fun). Frequently, a parent may have more success incorporating therapeutic ideas into regular family activities. For instance, mixing cookie dough with the hands provides a novel touch sensation. Allowing a child to pull taffy or chop vegetables (with careful supervision) may increase hand strength and dexterity.

Some useful suggestions for parents may include taking the children to different playgrounds in order to encourage interaction with new equipment, or planning family outings which include opportunities for heavy work activities. Children love to wrestle or horseplay with a parent who provides safe touch sensations. Bath time can provide opportunities for messy play or to experience different touch sensations such as washcloths, sponges, or gentle brushes. Bedtime may be a good time for deep-pressure stroking or massage which can help a child calm and prepare for a good night's sleep.

When we provide the information necessary for the parent to understand how their child "works," the parents can help the child get through difficult situations. Parents should be parents, giving unconditional love rather than attempting to be home therapists.

A Note to Parents

Parents of overaroused children frequently complain of how poor their child's behavior is following a school day. Home is a haven, a place to recover. In many instances, the child may "hold it together at school" only to have to "let it all out" when home. These children may be overaroused and need to find means to calm themselves. Your job as a parent therapist is to help your child find appropriate ways to become calm and regroup.

In any activity, be aware of your voice, body posture, and tension level. If you want to help your child to relax, use a slower, calm voice. If you feel tense, use a harsh or shrill voice, or move quickly, the child will have a more difficult time relaxing. Use your body, voice, and muscle tone to reflect the calmness you are trying to help the child obtain.

Giving Positive Support

One therapy story emphasizes the importance of positive, supportive parent involvement. Jason had been receiving therapy for about a year. He emphatically did not want his mother or father to participate or observe his therapy activities. At age 10, Jason had made significant progress in the areas of balance, eye-hand coordination, bilateral integration, and sequencing. One day Jason felt he had mastered a game which required him to hit a large therapy ball away from himself as he balanced on a rocker board. Jason asked his father to watch the game, and later he asked his father to throw the large ball. Jason challenged his dad to "Try to knock me off balance."

Jason's father accepted the challenge and succeeded in causing Jason to lose his balance and fall off the board. Jason was embarrassed and angry. However, he got back on the board to continue the game. Jason's father quickly succeeded in knocking him off again. At this time the therapist intervened. Needless to say, Jason did not ask his father to participate in his therapy sessions for a long time.

This incident suggests that Jason's father did not understand the concept of the "just-right challenge." Presenting the "just-right challenge" requires that children are presented with the correct amount of challenge to make them tax their skills while allowing them to complete the task successfully. Jason's father apparently did not understand that Jason was really asking his father to watch him succeed and help him win the game— not to really knock him off. Or perhaps Jason's father did not have good motor-control skills to accurately direct the amount of force he exerted on the ball. Regardless, parents, therapists, and teachers must help the child win. Children need to feel successful. As a child's skill develops and confidence improves, the activity may be restructured to allow the child to experience wins and losses in a safe environment.

Games for Home

Groundhog

This game involves allowing the child to crawl beneath the cushions on the couch, underneath a beanbag chair, or under a pile of blankets.

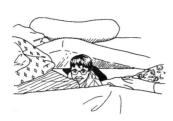

Implications: This activity provides equal weight to the whole body, which helps to tilt the seesaw toward calming. (See the illustration of the nervous system discussed on pages 56-57.)

Flashlight Tag

In a closet or darkened room, the child tags objects by directing a flashlight beam on them.

Some parents use this game to help their child practice spelling words. The child uses the beam of light to write the word on the ceiling. It may be best to have the child lie on the floor and look at the ceiling. This positioning may help to calm the child.

Implications: The darkness of the room, minimizing of visually stimulating input, and your calming voice all contribute to the calming effect of the game.

Burrito

The child lies on a sheet or lightweight blanket and is slowly rolled into it "like a burrito." The therapist parent can squeeze the burrito, if the child permits it.

A variation of the game is called Hot Dog. The child is rolled into a sheet or blanket, and the therapist parent pretends to apply "condiments," using different touches. The parent may "spread the ketchup" by rubbing the child from head to toes; or "add some cheese" by lightly squeezing the child. "Pickles" may be lightly tapped on.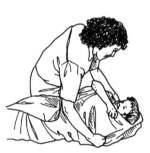

Implications: In this game, it is important for the child to feel in control. If the child feels confined, any calming effect is quickly eliminated. When the child is enjoying the game, the neutral warmth of the covers, deep-touch pressure, and your calming voice can facilitate the child's ability to calm.

Pillowcase

Encourage the child to "Get small enough to fit into a pillowcase." A smaller child may be able to fit inside an actual pillowcase. Ask a larger child to try to fit beneath the coffee table or into a cabinet.

Implications: Children with poor body schema or body size awareness can explore their bodies and see where they fit.

Therapeutic Activities

Obstacle Courses

Obstacle courses can be designed to be as simple as following a masking-tape path over a variety of objects, underneath chairs, around tight corners, and through barrels and hoops. If the setting permits, the obstacle course is a unique setup that stimulates the child to use previously learned

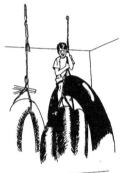

skills in new and different ways. Favorite obstacles include inclined bolsters, platform swings, rope ladders, and suspended ropes, trapezes, and inner tubes.

Implications: Obstacle courses can facilitate the development of bilateral integration, sequencing, timing, balance, and body awareness as well as promote improved motor planning.

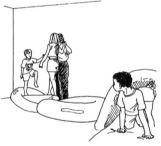
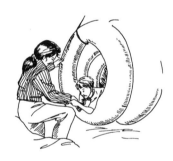

T-Stool Catch

The therapist and child sit on one-legged stools while playing catch. During the game, language and sequencing tasks can be added.

Another option is to have the therapist roll the ball to the child and require the child to stop the ball with a designated body part called out by the therapist. (For example, while throwing the ball, the therapist can call out, "Right foot" or "Left hand.") Varying the timing of the verbal cues makes the game more challenging.

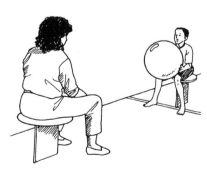

Implications: This game works on balance and eye-hand coordination. It can be modified to work on right/ left awareness or speech goals.

Popcorn*

This game requires a therapy ball at least 36 inches in diameter. The ball is pushed into a corner of the room, mats are placed in front of it, and 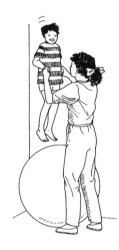 the therapist's body anchors the ball against the wall. The child climbs on top of the ball, securely holds the therapist's hands, and jumps as high as possible. The child can be asked to count, talk about the day, or alternate feet while continuing to jump.

Implications: Jumping facilitates the body's ability to feel the position of the muscles and joints (proprioception). Depending on the child, proprioception can be used to stimulate or calm the nervous system.

Incredible Hulk*

Theraband® is required to play this game. This wide elastic band comes in rolls of a few yards. If unavailable, an elastic bandage may be used. With the child's permission, the therapist wraps the child like a mummy. While on a mat surface, the child assumes various rolling, moving, and sitting postures. At the end of the game, the child breaks out of the elastic wrapping by pulling it over the body.

Implications: Using this tight wrapping facilitates body, muscle, and joint awareness. It also may calm an overaroused sense of touch. However, this game needs the child's permission because it can be threatening to some children.

---

*A child can be introduced to these less-pleasant activities, but should never be forced to participate in them.

Bird Seed*

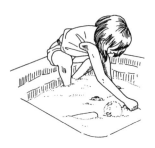

For this game, the child plays in a small, plastic wading pool filled with bird seed, sand, rice, or other dry material. The child may place hands, feet, arms, and legs into the material. The child feels for "buried treasure" (paper clips, small cars, coins, dice, rubber bands, buttons, and other small objects).

To make the game more challenging, the child can be blindfolded.

Implications: This game facilitates the development of discriminatory touch. The child who is overresponsive to touch sensations will probably not want to place hands or feet into this textured material. Gradually as the tactile system normalizes, the child will become more comfortable with these unusual sensations.

Big Foot*

The child is encouraged to fill large socks with bird seed or sand and then put them on. The child may walk in the large socks or navigate a course laid out by the therapist.

Implications: The texture provides touch input, while the weight of the socks provides deep-touch pressure and promotes awareness of body position.

Dodge Ball

This game is played using a scooterboard and a suspended swinging ball. The child lies prone on the scooterboard. The ball is pushed at a steady rhythm as the child attempts to propel the scooterboard in just the right timing to clear the ball before getting touched by it.

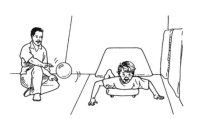

---

*A child can be introduced to these less-pleasant activities, but should never be forced to participate in them.

Implications: While working on timing and sequencing, the child is strengthening back and neck extensor muscles. This game also facilitates eye-hand coordination.

The Giant Tomato

The child lies prone on a scooterboard. The therapist pushes a large therapy ball behind the child, who is propelling the scooterboard toward a target. If the child reaches the target first, she wins. If the "giant tomato" catches the child, she is "slimed with ketchup" as the therapist gently pushes the ball over the child.

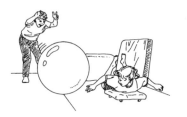

Implications: This activity combines the bilateral activity of propelling the scooterboard with the deep-touch pressure of the ball providing calming input for the child.

Scooterboard Hockey

This game requires two scooterboards, masking tape to mark boundaries, two cardboard bricks, and a ball. The object of the game is to hit the ball into the opponent's goal area. To hit the ball, both hands must be holding the cardboard brick.

Implications: Working in prone (on the stomach) is great for strengthening the back and neck muscles. This game also promotes eye-hand coordination. Keeping two hands on the brick to push the ball promotes both sides of the body working together. Maneuvering the scooterboard in such an awkward position increases the child's body awareness.

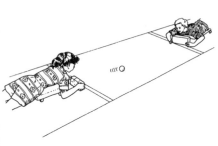

Top Gun*

If a suspended hammock swing is available, the child may swing in prone position as if flying. Targets are placed around the child. (We use cones 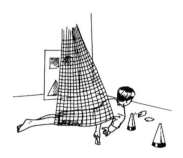 of red and white as targets.) The child tries to knock down the targets by throwing beanbags at them. The targets may be stacked to provide a more- or less-stable target, depending on the child's skill level.

Implications: This activity provides movement sensation while the child is flying in the net swing. This sensation promotes muscle tone, while the throwing activity encourages eye-hand coordination. The targets may be placed to require the child to cross midline while throwing the beanbags.

Whale*

While the child is swinging in a suspended hammock, the therapist pushes a large ball—"the whale"—into the child. The child may either dodge the whale or enjoy the sensation of having the whale crash into the net.

Implications: The pressure of the ball modulates the movement provided by the net swing. The ball pushing into the net causes a sudden change in direction, which increases the child's ability to perceive the change in the movement.

---

*Caution: This activity should not be implemented by teachers or parents.** Suspended equipment is frequently unavailable in the school environment due to safety issues. If suspended equipment is to be used, it must be well installed in order to support the weight of the child and the momentum created by the child's movement. Treatment using suspended equipment must be supervised by therapists trained in its use and well aware of contraindications such as sensory overload.

CHAPTER 6

Consultation

Occupational and physical therapists are frequently asked to evaluate and treat students in the school setting. Private therapists also may contribute to the evaluation and treatment process. Once the evaluation process is complete, appropriate treatment plans can be established. These plans may include private therapy, school-based therapy, or a combination of the two. Even within the school setting, services may include direct treatment or consultation. The therapist's role is to work with teachers and parents to provide the best possible program for each child.

The initial referral for evaluation may come from a variety of sources. Frequently, the classroom teacher is the first person to observe a child's behavior as compared to that of the child's peers. A teacher may notice a child having difficulty with organizational skills, thus struggling to complete assignments on time. A child who appears frustrated and distracted may be responding to demands that exceed the capabilities of an overstressed nervous system. A teacher observing these behaviors may initiate a referral to the school diagnostician or other appropriate personnel to begin the referral process to address the child's educationally related needs.

Parents may see an entirely different picture of their child at home. A child who works very hard to keep pace at school may come home fatigued, releasing frustration resulting from a difficult school day. A child who experiences anxiety toward school may complain of stomachaches or headaches. These complaints may warrant medical evaluation to rule out potential causes other than school-related problems. A physician, psychologist, or diagnostician may recommend a private therapist to address a wider range of problems which affect learning and behavior.

In any case, a coordinated approach must be considered in order to address the full range of difficulties a child may experience. There seem to be no formal "rules" about who should be the case manager or coordinator in addressing the multiple needs of a child with learning disability. Is medically based treatment the appropriate approach for this child, or should school-based programs address the problem from an educationally relevant perspective? Who is to determine the best approach? The answers to these questions may be as varied as the children experiencing the difficulties.

The issue of who should be in charge and who should be the one to identify the problem does not have a simple solution. In many cases, the parents take on the role as case manager for their child and become their child's advocate. Parents are frequently the ones who coordinate the medically prescribed treatment and private therapy recommendations with the teachers and school personnel. These proactive parents relay the problems reported in the learning situation to the appropriate medical personnel. In other cases, it may be the school diagnostician who guides the parents through the process of testing and options for treatment.

Private therapists may provide services which address medically and educationally related issues. Generally, the private therapist is contacted by the child's parent or physician to validate or elaborate upon previous testing.

Once the "problem areas" have been identified, the case manager or parent must decide which areas should be addressed. In order to receive services through the school, testing must establish a discrepancy between a child's intellectual potential and academic performance. The special education committee designs the plan for services. However, the school's area of service is limited to those "educationally relevant" needs which directly impact the child's classroom performance.

It is important for the case manager to remember that there are many outside options for providing help for a child with learning or attention deficits. By continually reassessing the child's performance and needs, other more medically related therapies can be added to an educationally guided program.

While school-based therapists may be limited in the services they provide, they may be uniquely positioned to interface among physicians, private therapists, and school settings. Many times, the school-based therapist can interpret the medical language and diagnoses for the educational personnel. Other times, a private therapist may address an issue of generalized low muscle tone, while the school therapist focuses on the specific issue of pencil grasp. The school therapist also may make recommendations to the teacher to help the child's functional performance in the classroom. For example, the therapist may suggest modifications such as handouts to decrease the child's need to copy assignments from the chalkboard, thus reducing effort and preventing fatigue.

Many private therapists contract to school districts for consultation services. The school therapist may rely on the private therapist for specific evaluations such as the *Sensory Integration and Praxis Tests*. Based on the evaluation results, the two therapists may develop a coordinated treatment program.

In the past, when a child was qualified to receive therapy services through the schools, the therapist automatically removed the child from the classroom for therapy sessions. More recently, therapists are staying with the child in the classroom. This proves to be especially helpful when the classroom contains a majority of children receiving special education services (learning lab, content mastery, or self-contained classrooms).

When consulting in a regular or "mainstreamed" class, the therapist's presence may be disruptive to the other students in the class. In these situations, the therapist and teacher may want to meet during another mutually convenient time to discuss problem situations. However, it is important for the therapist to spend time in the classroom to completely evaluate the child's "environment" for learning.

Improving handwriting is a common request for occupational therapy intervention. A consultation in the classroom may be helpful to the students and teacher. For example, many children with handwriting problems may be able to improve their skills through additional practice. Other children may have more than a handwriting problem. Their difficulties with writing may be due to poor sensory feedback, decreased postural control, weak muscles, and decreased dexterity. After assessing the child, the occupational therapist may be able to explain more clearly to the parents and teacher the cause of the child's handwriting difficulty. After understanding the roots of the problem, they may be able to incorporate new approaches into the child's usual classroom routines which will prove to be more beneficial to the child and the teacher.

Other times, the therapist may be called upon for less usual tasks. The occupational and physical therapist are appropriate consultants to assess and remedy wheelchair accessibility issues. The recent revisions to the Consumer Product Safety Commission recommendations for playground safety have prompted many schools to replace their old, unsafe equipment. Occupational and physical therapists are able to help redesign a playground that is more "learning-disability friendly." The design might include areas of the playground for physical exertion for an overaroused child to vent extra energy. Other areas of the playground would include smaller, calmer places for the child to tune out some of the noise. Manufacturers offer many equipment options that can help to create an appropriate play environment that allows children to modulate their nervous systems.

Case Studies

The following case studies demonstrate how medical personnel, therapists, and the school personnel can all coordinate their efforts in the best interest of the child.

Although Jenny had no specific medical diagnosis other than low muscle tone, her physician insisted that she obtain speech and occupational therapy as part of her first grade school day. Jenny's occupational therapy evaluation showed lags of up to 30 months in gross motor and fine motor development. Although her receptive language tests were within the normal limits, her expressive language scores were significantly delayed because of her poor articulation. Jenny was socially aware, and during first grade seemed to enjoy being singled out of her class for special times in Occupational Therapy and Speech.

But during second grade, she resented being "pulled" out of class. Although her test scores had not improved enough for the special education committee to dismiss her from OT and Speech, occupational therapy services were modified to classroom consultations without direct therapy. The occupational therapist participated in classroom activities to help the teacher ease Jenny's fine motor requirements, suggested various seating arrangements, and set up "games" for Jenny to play when she had free time in her classroom. Jenny's teacher frequently remarked that the classroom consultations were helpful. In addition to learning new ways to help Jenny succeed in the classroom, the teacher had increased her knowledge base as she helped other children in the room. As the teacher increased her understanding of how Jenny "worked," teaching her seemed easier and was more successful.

Dillon attended school in a rural district. In class, he displayed learning difficulties which his parents believed had a sensory-integrative basis. They contacted a private therapist several hundred miles away who was certified in administering and interpreting the *Sensory Integration and Praxis Tests.* They were able to arrange for their local school district to pay for the evaluation and appropriate treatment plan. On a two-day trip to the city, they consulted with a pediatric neurologist, a developmental optometrist, and the occupational therapist who administered the SIPT battery. The test results and interpretation were mailed to the parents, and a phone conference followed. Because of the parent's efforts, Dillon was able to receive an appropriate therapy program which combined private therapy and school-based services.

After receiving approximately two years of service in his local district, Dillon returned to the city for a follow-up evaluation. His reevaluation revealed significant gains in all areas assessed and pointed to the refining of his treatment program to address the remaining deficits in a more specific manner. Ongoing consultation consisted of occasional phone calls from the school-based therapist or parents to address specific problem areas.

Summary

The occupational therapist has an important role to play with children who have learning disabilities. An evaluation can point to the cause of the child's problem and frequently to a solution. Even when no satisfactory solution is available, the therapist can provide information to the teacher and parent which can help the child function more successfully in the school environment. Private and school-based therapists often work together to plan and carry out an appropriate treatment program for each child. Learning disabilities and attention problems do not just disappear as the child matures; but with proper evaluation and remediation, the effects of the disability can be minimized. An effective treatment program seeks to remediate the child's deficits, make indicated changes in the environment, and provide information to teachers and parents in order to maximize the child's potential to succeed.

CHAPTER 7

Case Studies

This chapter contains eight in-depth studies of clinical cases, including evaluation results, treatment activities, and outcomes. They serve to illustrate a variety of problems and intervention strategies. They have been selected based on their ability to contribute to the understanding of the therapy process.

Case Study Index

The following synopsis of each case study is provided so that readers may easily identify the main points and select cases which most nearly address their individual interests.

Case Study #1—Manuel

Manuel was identified at age 6 by his preschool teacher, who had noted poor gross and fine motor skills. His parents also were concerned about aggressive behavior. His initial evaluation revealed poor processing of movement sensations as well as extreme hypersensitivity to touch. His therapy program extended over a 3½-year period and was highly successful in addressing both the motor and behavior issues.

Case Study #2—Bonnie

Bonnie was referred for an occupational therapy evaluation at age 11. She was initially referred for therapy because of her visual-perception problems. Testing revealed severe motor development lags. During her course of occupational therapy, additional educational testing confirmed definite right-hemisphere learning disabilities.

Case Study #3—Eduard

Eduard was screened by occupational therapists at his private school. His teachers suspected that sensorimotor problems were contributing to his learning and behavior problems. He did not receive treatment until two years later. His case illustrates how sensory-processing problems can affect a child and his ability to learn and socialize.

Case Study #4—Lorrie

Lorrie had been evaluated by a neurologist at 23 months and received a diagnosis of "mild hypotonia." On a follow-up evaluation by the neurologist at age 6, she received a diagnosis of attention deficit disorder. Shortly after, she began intensive tutoring and perceptual therapies. At age 8, occupational therapy evaluations were requested by her tutors to help understand more clearly the difficulties Lorrie was experiencing.

Case Study #5—Emily

Emily was first seen at 3 years of age due to delayed speech and motor skills. The *Miller Assessment for Preschoolers* (Miller 1988) indicated a need for treatment. She received occupational therapy and speech therapy for three years, and later was enrolled in a school for children with language and learning delays.

Case Study #6—Brady

Brady was referred by a family therapist for an evaluation of sensory integration based on extremely aggressive behavior. His evaluation showed extremely aversive responses to touch and underresponsiveness to movement. His therapy program helped him to achieve a calmer state and improved his behavior and school performance.

Case Study #7—Jonathan

Jonathan had a complex medical history, including episodes of stoppage of breathing as an infant, severe ear infections, and a head trauma at age 3. He was referred by the hospital to an occupational therapist for evaluation and treatment. Through his therapy program, he gained skills in motor planning, became increasingly physically active, and showed gains in self-confidence.

Case Study #8—Sarah

Sarah was a frail child with no significant medical history, but she showed delays in speech and low muscle tone which adversely affected her motor development. She received private occupational therapy in addition to occupational therapy and speech services at school. Her therapy program resulted in improved muscle tone, increased strength, and gains in gross motor and fine motor skills. She emerged from a shy, insecure first grader to a happy, socially adept young lady.

Case Study #1—Manuel

This 6-year-old boy was referred to occupational therapy by his private preschool for delayed gross motor and fine motor skills. According to the parent questionnaire, aggressive behavior was an additional concern. His medical history was unremarkable except for a history of ear infections, which necessitated the insertion of pressure-equalizing tubes at the age of 2. He attended a small private school that specialized in the early treatment of speech and language delays.

The occupational therapy evaluation consisted of administration of the *Southern California Sensory Integration Tests* (Ayres 1972) in addition to clinical observations of eye and hand usage, postural responses, and other neuromuscular conditions relating to behavior and learning.

The evaluation identified deficits in processing movement and touch sensations, resulting in poor gross and fine motor developmental and tactual defensiveness (hypersensitivity to touch sensations). His therapy program was designed to provide opportunities such as spinning and swinging in a net swing and other suspended equipment. The touch issues were to be addressed through a desensitization program involving presentation of a variety of textures and touch sensations. Gross motor skills were facilitated by providing a variety of therapy activities such as scooterboard games and suspended obstacle courses. Fine motor activities included manipulative activities such as puzzles, games, and arts and crafts.

During initial treatment sessions, it became clear that Manuel was easily overwhelmed by sensory stimuli. He reacted to the therapist's attempts to engage him in therapeutic activities by hitting, kicking, and biting. The therapist revised the therapy program to include activities designed to calm an overaroused nervous system. These included deep-pressure activities such as hiding under therapy mats.

Manuel frequently came into therapy as a specific animal. These included a cockroach, a hermit crab, and a tiger. The therapist suggested a nest or den appropriate to the animal. These were constructed of bolsters or tires and therapy mats. Manuel was encouraged to come out of his nest to play on the equipment for short times before retreating to his habitat. Initial activities were one-dimensional, such as climbing a bolster hung at one end to form a "mountain." As Manuel's skill and confidence grew, the activities became more complex, involving transfers between pieces of therapy equipment.

As Manuel's nervous system became more resilient, he was encouraged to engage in more intense movement activities. He often spent the majority of his 30-minute treatment sessions with intense spinning in a therapy net. As his nervous system slowly normalized, his desire for spinning and swinging decreased and he began to seek out more developmentally mature activities. Touch sensitivity remained a problem area, causing him to resist activities such as locating coins embedded in bird seed or—worse yet—finger painting. His disordered touch system also caused him to have difficulty in situations in which he might inadvertently be touched by another child. His mother reported that he had difficulty standing in line and frequently showed aggressive behavior on the playground. Therapeutic brushing techniques and deep-touch pressure such as stroking were used to desensitize his overly responsive sense of touch.

Manuel's therapy program covered a period of 3½ years. Periodic reevaluations were conducted to measure change over time. These reevaluations consisted of the Bruininks-Oseretsky *Test of Motor Proficiency* (Bruininks 1978), the *Developmental Test of Visual-Motor Integration* (Beery and Buktenica 1989), and the Postrotary Nystagmus Subtest of the SIPT (Ayres 1989). Throughout his treatment program, Manuel showed gains in gross and fine motor skill development. During the course of his treatment, he was placed on Ritalin due to an identified attention deficit. He also received psychological intervention aimed at helping him to articulate his feelings and modulate his stress. His occupational therapy program addressed the identified stress through engagement in activities such as slow spinning in the net or nestling in the mats. He also showed improved social skills, as evidenced by his ability to interact with other children in games and contests.

Toward the end of his therapy program, the therapist suggested appropriate transitional activities for Manuel. He joined a swim program and Cub Scouts. Manuel eventually left the sheltered environment of the private school and entered a public school program in which he tested for and was placed in the academically gifted program. No follow-up services were recommended.

One of the therapist's fondest memories of Manuel was the day he entered his treatment session announcing that he wasn't an animal any more. He was a cowboy!

Case Study #2—Bonnie

Bonnie was referred for private occupational therapy testing by her developmental optometrist and her educational tutor. She attended her neighborhood public school and had repeated second grade. At age 11, fourth grade was becoming increasingly difficult. Her primary problems were thought to be in the areas of visual perception. However, testing using the *Southern California Sensory Integration Tests* (Ayres 1972) revealed that Bonnie also had problems in areas relating to how her body was able to process information about movement (vestibular processing), accurately interpret touch information (tactile discrimination), and coordinate her body to perform new movement activities (motor planning).

Initial testing using the Bruininks-Oseretsky *Test of Motor Proficiency* (Bruininks 1978) gave her an age-equivalent gross motor score of 8 years, 11 months and a fine motor score of 8 years, 2 months. Her balance score was in the 6-year range. (See page 86 for Bonnie's testing results on the Bruininks-Oseretsky *Test of Motor Proficiency.*) During her course of therapy, the Beery-Buktenica *Developmental Test of Visual-Motor Integration* (1989) also was performed. (See page 84 for the results of her testing on the Beery-Buktenica *Developmental Test of Visual-Motor Integration.*)

Initially, Bonnie's therapy sessions were scheduled twice weekly for 30 minutes. The majority of these sessions was spent involved in movement-related (vestibular) activities, including eye-hand coordination. A typical game involved Bonnie swinging on her stomach in the suspended therapy net as she tossed beanbags into various targets. Gross motor balance activities involved obstacle courses. Bonnie's movements were usually slow and carefully planned. She seemed to have to think about how her body needed to move. As her scores began to normalize, therapy was modified to weekly sessions of 60 minutes. These 60-minute sessions included 30 minutes of more gross motor activities followed by fine motor, perceptual, and sequencing activities.

Her mother was concerned about Bonnie's ability to socialize with peers. Bonnie was tall and mature-looking for her age. Her poor motor skills and slow speech made it difficult for her to be accepted by her peers. During the course of therapy, Bonnie's mother commented about how Bonnie seemed to be getting increased confidence and was beginning to be invited to other girls' homes for parties.

As junior high approached, her parents pursued additional educational testing. This testing confirmed definite learning disabilities relating to the right cerebral hemisphere of the brain. The evaluator made private-school recommendations. Bonnie's educational program was tailored to her diagnosed learning difficulties and strengths. Occupational therapy and tutoring were gradually decreased.

During one conference, Bonnie's parents expressed their happiness over how Bonnie had improved the speed and accuracy of her handwriting, how she had improved her balancing, and how her confidence had increased. Although her motor-performance scores might never catch up to those of her peers, they believed that Bonnie had made tremendous progress. We discussed discharge and possible areas to investigate to continue to help Bonnie. Her father stated, "At some point in time we must decide when to quit trying to fix what may never be right with Bonnie and begin to accentuate all of the things she is good at doing." As she continued therapy and tutoring services, her teachers, therapists, and parents investigated art classes and choir groups to begin to accentuate her positives. Gradually she was discharged from Occupational Therapy. She continued to receive tutoring for her school work.

During a phone conference a year after Bonnie's discharge from private OT, her mother reported she was keeping up her grades during her freshman year in high school. Bonnie was taking the modified-level classes recommended by her counselors. She was able to take an art class in school, and was thoroughly enjoying taking additional classes at a private art institute.

On her 6- and 12-month follow-up evaluations, Bonnie showed slight improvements on some of her Beery-Buktenica fine motor subtests, and she had maintained her skill levels as measured by the Bruininks-Oseretsky test. (See pages 84-85 for the results of Bonnie's retesting on the Beery-Buktenica *Developmental Test of Visual-Motor Integration;* and page 86 for her retesting results on the Bruininks-Oseretsky *Test of Motor Proficiency.*)

Excerpts from Bonnie's Initial Test Results Beery-Buktenica *Developmental Test of Visual-Motor Integration*

Chronological Age: 12 years

VMI Raw Score: 16

VMI Age Equivalent: 8 years, 7 months

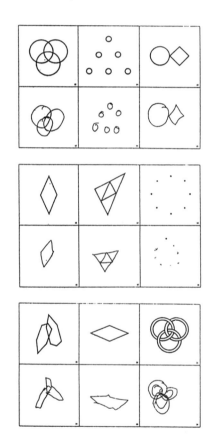

Excerpts from Bonnie's Retesting Results
Beery-Buktenica *Developmental Test of Visual-Motor Integration*

Chronological Age: 13 years, 3 months

VMI Raw Score: 20

VMI Age Equivalent: 12 years, 7 months

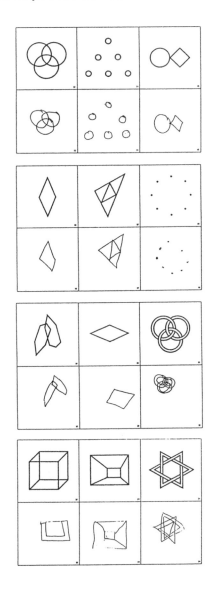

Bonnie's Summary of Reevaluations
Bruininks-Oseretsky *Test of Motor Proficiency*

Occupational Therapy Center, Inc.
2500 Tanglewilde, Suite 330
Houston, Texas 77063

Summary of Reevaluations

Name: Bonnie

Test Administered: BRUININKS-OSERETSKY TEST OF
MOTOR PROFICIENCY

Date Tested: Chronological Age:	6-93 11 yr 2 mo	12-93 11 yr 8 mo	9-94 12 yr 5 mo
Running Speed and Agility	8-0	8-11	8-11
Balance	6-5	8-11	10-2
Bilateral Coordination	8-8	9-5	
Strength	7-2	7-11	
Upper-Limb Coordination		8-5	
Response Speed	5-8	8-11	8-11
Visual-Motor		9-2	
Upper-Limb Speed and Dexterity	8-2	8-2	11-2

Scores on this summary chart are reported in age equivalency. For example,
5-8 means the child is performing the items on the subtest similarly to a child
age 5 years, 8 months.

Please refer to the attached report for specifics on scores.

Case Study #3—Eduard

Eduard's private school annually requested therapists from a private clinic to screen children attending their school. The teachers recommended children for screening. With the parents' consent, two therapists completed brief evaluations on the children. The screening was designed to see if in-depth testing for sensorimotor problems was indicated. The screening included clinical observation of balance, hopping, antigravity postures, eye movements, copying simple geometric designs, and the child's responses to movement on a large therapy ball and a slow spinning activity.

Eduard was initially screened at age 6 years, 11 months. His screening showed decreased hand strength, inability to quickly imitate body postures, poor eye movements, and decreased muscle strength for holding prone and supine positions. His ability to process movement information (Postrotary Nystagmus Subtest on the SIPT; Ayres 1989) scored below the average range. He scored in the bottom range, 2%, on the *Riley Motor Problems Inventory* (Riley 1972). Eduard was recommended for further testing.

His parents pursued more complete sensorimotor testing. The *Sensory Integration and Praxis Tests* (Ayres 1989) confirmed sensorimotor problems in the areas of processing of movement information (vestibular processing), touch reception (poor discrimination and tactile defensiveness), decreased balance, poor eye-hand coordination, and motor-planning deficits. Because of difficulties in obtaining insurance reimbursement for occupational therapy services, Eduard did not receive any therapy.

A year passed, and Eduard again was recommended for screening by his teachers. As he entered the screening room, Eduard dragged his feet as he walked, looked down at the floor, and generally appeared "shut down." When asked to perform different activities, he shrugged his shoulders and said, "I'll try, but I don't think I can do that." His screening scores were generally lower than those of his initial screening, with the most significant drop in fine motor performance.

After another 12 months of trying unsuccessfully to obtain insurance reimbursement, Eduard's parents decided to begin therapy using their own finances. When Eduard first came to therapy, he was very quiet and withdrawn. His therapist provided many opportunities to arouse his nervous system. Initially, he gravitated toward intense movement activities such as spinning and swinging. He had difficulty climbing on therapy equipment, and he quickly gave up when tasks were difficult for him.

Slowly he began to improve in his skills and gain self-confidence. He increased eye contact and became more positive in his approach to unfamiliar tasks. His parents noted the increased confidence and were able to follow the therapist's suggestions to help him be more organized at school and at home. Unfortunately, they decided to discontinue therapy after only four months because of financial constraints. The therapist encouraged them to continue, fearing that Eduard would quickly lose the gains he had made and that his self-esteem would suffer.

Eduard never returned to therapy. At the next annual screening at school, his teacher reported that he was having definite difficulty keeping pace with his classmates. Handwriting was tedious for him, and he was slow to complete his assignments. He had made few friends that year and had become increasingly withdrawn. His parents had become frustrated with his lack of progress and were considering enrolling him in public school so that he could get special education services.

Case Study #4—Lorrie

This pleasant 8-year-old girl was referred for sensorimotor testing to provide additional information to her parents and tutor about why she was continuing to have so many difficulties with school and learning. Her complete *Sensory Integration and Praxis Tests* (SIPT) evaluation is included to show how much information can be obtained from the SIPT. Also included are descriptions of her therapy regime and her 12-month re-evaluation.

Occupational Therapy Center, Inc.
2500 Tanglewilde, Suite 330
Houston, Texas 77063

Occupational Therapy Initial Evaluation

Name: Lorrie _____
Birth Date: April 12, 1986
Test Date: June 4, 1994
Chronological Age: 8 Years, 2 Months

Referral Source: Mrs. _____, Perceptual Education Therapy. Mrs. _____ has been working with Lorrie since January, 1994. Mrs. _____ reports Lorrie has made good progress, but she felt this evaluation would provide further insight into Lorrie's difficulties.

Test Administered: Sensory Integration and Praxis Tests (SIPT) Clinical Observations including eye-hand usage, postural responses, muscle tone, and other neurological indicators of behavior and learning.

Test Results: Please refer to the attached handouts for detailed explanation of the tests administered and scores. The tests were administered during two sessions, each lasting approximately one hour. Lorrie was rather quiet during the seated portions of the SIPT, but became more talkative during the gross motor and clinical portions. She attended well, cooperated for all of the subtests, and did not appear to become frustrated as the tests became more challenging. These test results should be considered accurate within the intrinsic reliability of the tests themselves.

Scores are expressed in Standard Deviation form. (-1.0 to +1.0 is considered in the average range.) Lorrie's scores were widely scattered, with relative strength areas in those areas requiring minimal motor response. Her lower scores were in those areas requiring tactile discrimination and localization, balance, bilateral movement, and motor planning. The following paragraphs will review her individual test performance.

The initial test administered was Space Visualization. Here the child must complete a formboard by first visually imagining the correct answer, followed by actually moving the block. Her performance was -1.7 S.D. The Figure-Ground subtest is another visual-perception test with minimal movement requirements. Lorrie's score was -0.8 S.D. a low-average score.

Lorrie's tactile (touch) system tests were primarily in the deficit range. Those tests included: Manual Form Perception, Kinesthesia, Finger Identification, Graphesthesia, and Localization of Tactile Stimuli. All of these subtests were performed with vision occluded. Her low scores suggest that touch perception may not be functioning to its potential. For example, Lorrie had difficulty identifying the shapes of objects in her hand to match with others on the Manual Form Perception subtest. This performance may relate either to difficulty coordinating two sides of her body or to poor tactile discrimination. The Kinesthesia subtest required Lorrie to return her arm to a previously marked place. Her inability to accurately retrace the motion may suggest her poor ability to know where her arm is if she cannot visually monitor it. Her scores on the subtests requiring her to point to which finger was touched and to put her finger exactly on the spot on her arm that was touched also were in the deficit range. Her better performance was on the Graphesthesia subtest, where Lorrie was able to retrace shapes drawn on the back of her hand.

The motor-planning subtests evaluate a child's ability to perform a new, unlearned movement pattern from either verbal or visual cues. Those subtests included: Praxis on Verbal Command, Design Copying, Constructional Praxis, Postural Praxis, and Oral Praxis. Lorrie's best performance in this area was on the Praxis on Verbal Command Subtest, where the child is required to perform physical actions to verbal cues. Her performance score was +0.2 S.D., but her time score was -1.3 S.D. This suggests that she has the verbal skills to perform the tasks, but she moves more slowly in response to those verbal instructions. She also was slow in copying the examiner's movements on the Postural Praxis Subtest. This slowness can be somewhat attributed to her poor sensory feedback, noted by her poor performance on the tactile tests. Lorrie had difficulty building the three-dimensional block structure on Constructional Praxis. This poor performance could be related to poor visual-perception of the required task, or poor sequencing, or ideation on where or how to begin. Her Sequencing Praxis score reflects her inability to repeat more than a three-step series of hand postures and inability to individually sequence her fingers.

Lorrie also showed difficulty with coordinating the two body sides; they seemed to work independently of each other, as observed in her attempting to repeat rhythmic arm motions. One side moved and then the other; they did not move in a smooth, coordinated manner. Poor bilateral coordination also affects balance and new motor planning. Theoretically, the body-extremity motions provide a view of how the two cerebral hemispheres communicate. Lorrie may not be able to utilize right- and left-brain information in a smooth, coordinated manner.

Lorrie performed in the deficit range on the Standing and Walking Balance Subtest. For example, Lorrie was able to balance on one foot with her eyes closed for a maximum of two seconds. It took Lorrie three attempts to correctly heel-to-toe walk.

She met the test requirements for the Motor Accuracy Subtest, which requires the child to trace a curved line. Her performance on this test when compared to the Design Copying fine motor test suggests she has sufficient fine motor pencil control to trace a simple line. However, the additional requirement of redrawing a visual-perception stimulus appeared difficult for her. Her Design Copying score was -0.8 S.D. Lorrie showed perceptual and se-quencing errors more frequently than fine motor control errors.

The Postrotary Nystagmus Subtest of the SIPT is one method of assessing how the vestibular system responds to movement and gravity. This relatively discrete vestibular-ocular reflex is one in-dicator of how well sensory information is processed and relayed through the midbrain. Lorrie enjoyed the rotation. Her low score suggests that vestibular information may not be adequately re-layed from the semicircular canals in the ear through the brain-stem to the eyes. Other clinical indicators of the vestibular system integrity substantiated this as an immature area for Lorrie. Those observations included:

Prone extension	Below average
Muscle co-contraction	Below average
Supine flexion	Below average

Impression: Lorrie appears to have numerous sensory processing deficits that may be related to or contributing to her reported dif-ficulties in visual perception. Her parents were kind in sharing previous evaluations of her developmental optometrist, neurolo-gist, diagnostician, and tutor.

In previous tests, Lorrie has shown tendencies toward low muscle tone, poor ability to follow directions, completing her work too slowly, poor gross motor skills, and making letter reversals. Her mother completed our Parent Questionnaire, which revealed Lorrie's difficulty with buttoning, not riding a tricycle until age 5, still using training wheels for her two-wheeler, and being "fearful" on higher playground equipment. Although these tendencies can be seen in "normal" and "learning disabled" children, Lorrie's test results suggest some of these difficulties may be related to immature sensory processing.

Theoretically, the tactile and vestibular neurological systems assist the other neurological systems in maturation and processing. Lorrie's touch and movement systems do not appear to be providing her with a good foundation from which to mature. When these neurological systems are not functioning adequately, dysfunctions occur in the "end-products" of our motor skills. This seems to be true for Lorrie; her balance, coordination of the two body sides, motor-planning abilities, and fine motor and gross motor skills are all performed below the levels typical for her age.

Lorrie seems to be having difficulties with motor-planning new tasks. The tendency to have difficulties in this area is termed *dyspraxia*. Poor motor planning may evidence itself in poor gross motor coordination, letter reversals, and slow work pace. A child with dyspraxia must "think through" movements that should be automatic. For example, this child may have to think through the series of motions to get each letter turned in the correct direction. Consequently, she is slow at completing work.

Poor tactile feedback also will slow one's rate of work. Lorrie may have to visually direct how she writes. The Kinesthesia Subtest suggests that she does not have a good sense of arm position. Poor tactile feedback also may evidence itself in appearing clumsy or awkward because one may not be able to "feel" where the body is in relationship to the surroundings. Theoretically, the tactile system contributes to the maturation of the visual cortex. Consequently, a child who has had less than optimum tactile information may have difficulty with accurate visual interpretation.

The Postrotary Nystagmus Subtest is one indicator of the efficiency of the movement system. Lorrie's score suggested low-average response. Additional clinical indicators of the movement system's immaturity include her poor balance, lower muscle tone, slowed rate of speech, and poor ability to hold and maintain postures that require antigravity muscle strength. Her previously reported fearfulness on playground equipment may be related to an immature movement system, and too much motion in the wrong direction may have felt uncomfortable for her.

Lorrie's poor bilateral integration affects gross motor and fine motor skill performance. Her poor bilateral coordination may have negatively affected her performance on Sequencing Praxis. However, Lorrie has shown tendencies toward poor sequencing, which can be seen in her poor ability to put pictures in the correct order, follow three- or four-step commands, or recall a motor sequence such as a new game in P.E. Poor sequencing skills also may contribute to her slow, labored writing. Buttoning requires good bilateral coordination and sequencing. If there is difficulty with either aspect, buttoning will be difficult.

Summary: Lorrie's SIPT test results suggest that her poorer processing of tactile and vestibular information may be contributing to her reported visual-perceptual deficits. This testing suggests that poor tactile feedback, poor bilateral coordination, poor vestibular processing, and poor motor planning also are contributing to Lorrie's previously diagnosed Mixed Specific Developmental Disorder.

Recommendations: Private occupational therapy is recommended to assist in further maturation of those underlying neurological conditions. Although Lorrie may have specific learning and visual-perceptual deficits, it is this therapist's opinion that by improving Lorrie's "foundation" for learning, we may improve her tactile feedback and motor planning and decrease the effort currently required for gross motor and fine motor performance. Therapy is recommended on a twice-weekly basis for 30-minute sessions. Specific goals will be established prior to the initiation of therapy. Prognosis for positive change is considered good. Formal reevaluation three months after beginning therapy.

Kathryn Miesner, OTR
Licensed Occupational Therapist

Therapy Regime

Lorrie attended occupational therapy sessions prior to her tutoring and vision therapy. Her therapy program emphasized working with both sides of her body simultaneously. She especially enjoyed the Popcorn activity (bouncing on a larger therapy ball; see page 67), and the therapist was able to feel how her arms had difficulty working together. Initially, Lorrie resisted movement activities; she preferred games incorporating more deep-touch pressure and body awareness. After approximately six months of therapy, she began attempting two- and three-step suspended obstacle courses. Her dyspraxia became very apparent when a climbing-and-balancing task that had been mastered one day would not be carried over if some of the components of the obstacle course were altered. Rather than frustrating herself, Lorrie attempted to perseverate on a course she had performed previously.

The majority of Lorrie's therapy time during her first year of therapy was centered around activities that reinforce body awareness and improve touch sensations (proprioception, kinesthesia, and decreasing tactile defensiveness). Significant progress was noted in her fine motor performance. By improving her total body foundation for performance, fine motor skills also improved.

Reevaluation

Lorrie was briefly retested three months after beginning therapy, using portions of the Bruininks-Oseretsky *Test of Motor Proficiency*. A complete reevaluation using the Bruininks-Oseretsky was performed six months after beginning occupational therapy. The report that follows reviews her progress 12 months after initiation of therapy. A summary chart of her performance on the Bruininks-Oseretsky test also is included.

Occupational Therapy Center, Inc.
2500 Tanglewilde, Suite 330
Houston, TX 77063

Occupational Therapy Reevaluation

Name: Lorrie _____
Birth Date: April 12, 1986
Test Date: July 9, 1995
Chronological Age: 9 Years, 3 Months
Tests Administered for this Reevaluation:
Bruininks-Oseretsky Test of Motor Proficiency
Southern California Sensory Integration Test (SCSIT) subtests
Clinical Observations

Reevaluation Results: Please refer to the attached summary of Lorrie's Bruininks score since her initial testing. The following portions of the Bruininks-Oseretsky subtests were readministered:

Running Speed and Agility. This subtest requires the child to run, retrieve a small object, and return. Score is obtained by performance time. Lorrie's time increased slightly above her reevaluation nine months ago to 5 years, 5 months.

Balance. Lorrie showed increases in her ability to balance on one foot with her eyes open. In October, 1994, she was able to balance on the beam for three seconds, which now has increased to eight seconds. She also has increased her ability to walk heel-to-toe on a tape line to six consecutive steps. However, she is unable to walk heel-to-toe on a balance beam.

Bilateral Coordination. This subtest observes ipsilateral (same side) and contralateral (alternating) arm and leg motions. Lorrie's performance remained consistent with her previous performance.

The Strength Subtest was performed when Lorrie's chronological age was 8 years, 6 months and her skill level equivalent was 5 years, 8 months. For this reevaluation, she scored in the 6 year, 8 month performance level; she increased her performance on sit-ups, push-ups and broad jump.

Upper-Limb Coordination. This subtest assesses eye-hand coordination using a tennis-sized ball. Finger coordination items also are observed. Lorrie's performance also increased on this subtest; she was able to bounce and catch the ball on three of five trials. In October she succeeded on one of five attempts.

Response Speed. Lorrie's performance on this quick eye-hand response test improved significantly. In October, she was unable to isolate her thumb to perform this task. Her performance on the subtest on this retesting increased to the 5 year, 8 month level.

Visual-Motor Control. In October, Lorrie's performance on this subtest was in the 7 year, 11 month range. Her performance on this reevaluation decreased slightly because she was less accurate on one of three drawings. However, her performance on the other two was similar to the previous testing, despite an increase in performance time.

Testing Performed	Time
6-94	65 seconds
10-94	45 seconds
7-95	22 seconds

Upper-Limb Speed and Dexterity. Lorrie's fine motor speed increases were also noted on this subtest. She manipulated pennies and cards faster and was able to make more pencil marks. Her age-equivalency time increased to the 6 year, 5 month level.

When Lorrie was initially evaluated, she was tested using the Sensory Integration and Praxis Tests (SIPT). For reevaluation, two subtests were repeated. They were scored using the criteria for the SIPT's predecessor, the Southern California Sensory Integration Tests (SCSIT).

Please recall that these scores are not statistically accurate for retest, but were readministered for a general comparison of skill levels. A score between -1.0 and +1.0 Standard Deviations (S.D.) is considered "average."

Kinesthesia. In this subtest, the child is asked to move her hand to a previously indicated position to assess how well she is able to "feel" where the arm is when she cannot visually monitor the motion. On the original SIPT, Lorrie's score was -2.7 S.D. On the retesting, her performance improved significantly to the +0.4 S.D. level. This suggests that Lorrie has increased her ability to know how her arm is moving without visually monitoring its motion.

Postrotary Nystagmus Subtest (PRN). This test assesses the movement (vestibular) system's responses to motion. The vestibular system assists with balance and is theorized to contribute to overall neurological maturation. On Lorrie's initial tests, her scores were in the dysfunctional range (-0.6 S.D.). Her retesting showed improvement in the processing of vestibular information with a score of -0.3 S.D. This is significant because her PRN score had not shown significant changes at the time of her last testing.

Clinically, Lorrie continues to improve her "foundational" skills. For example, she is able to motor plan to move on and off equipment with greater control. She is able to work in a prone position for up to eight minutes without displaying neck extensor muscle fatigue. Lorrie is beginning to climb and maneuver on higher surfaces, but occasionally exhibits a response that suggests these activities are too challenging for her.

Summary: Lorrie continues to make good progress in all areas tested. Her gross motor testing suggested increases in her skills of 6 to 12 months in this last nine-month period. She continues to make gains in gross motor coordination. Lorrie's dyspraxia (poor or slower motor planning) is still observed clinically, but has improved (as noted by previous retesting).

Tests repeated from her initial testing suggest her "foundation" for learning and coordination is improving. Her ability to know where her arm is will facilitate further fine motor progress. The measurable increase in her upper-arm kinesthesia is theorized to suggest that kinesthesia in her legs also is improving. Her vestibular system responses also are encouraging.

Recommendations: Occupational therapy is recommended to continue, with sessions scheduled twice weekly. Lorrie's therapy plan will be modified to reflect the changes noted in the reevaluation. Reevaluation in six to nine months.

Because Lorrie will be changing schools, I will assist with helping her new teachers to learn Lorrie's strengths and weaknesses, as requested.

Kathryn Miesner, OTR
Licensed Occupational Therapist

Lorrie's Summary of Reevaluations
Bruininks-Oseretsky *Test of Motor Proficiency*

Occupational Therapy Center, Inc.
2500 Tanglewilde, Suite 330
Houston, Texas 77063

Summary of Reevaluations

Name: Lorrie

Test Administered: BRUININKS-OSERETSKY TEST OF
MOTOR PROFICIENCY

Date Tested: Chronological Age:	6-94 8 yr 3 mo	12-94 8 yr 6 mo	9-95 9 yr 3 mo
Running Speed and Agility		4-11	5-5
Balance	4-2	4-11	5-8
Bilateral Coordination		5-11	5-11
Strength		5-8	6-8
Upper-Limb Coordination		4-11	5-8
Response Speed		< 4-2	5-8
Visual-Motor	6-8	7-11	7-5
Upper-Limb Speed and Dexterity	5-8	5-8	6-5

Scores on this summary chart are reported in age equivalency. For example, 5-8 means the child is performing the items on the subtest similarly to a child age 5 years, 8 months.

Please refer to the attached report for specifics on scores.

Continued Therapy Regime

During the continued course of therapy, her parents noted positive changes in Lorrie. Her father stated that Lorrie seemed to have more good days than bad days, as measured by how she greeted him when he came home from work. Her father was also pleasantly surprised by her recent interest in the neighborhood playground. She had been attending her church's school, but her parents and teachers felt that her educational needs were not being met. Lorrie began to attend a local school that specialized in teaching children with learning disabilities.

After approximately 24 months of therapy, Lorrie's sessions were decreased to once a week, and then to twice a month. Academically, she continued to struggle. At age 10, her gross motor skills plateaued in the 6-year age level. Her fine motor skills were in the 7-year range. Despite her poor motor skills, her attitude toward trying new activities and self-confidence were noticeably improved. At the time of discharge, her parents reiterated that they felt the combination of vision therapy, tutoring, occupational therapy, and her new private school had made a big difference in Lorrie's abilities. Their only regret is that they had not begun the intense therapy regime when they first discovered Lorrie was not performing at age-appropriate levels.

Case Study #5—Emily

Emily, age 3 years, 3 months, was referred to occupational therapy specifically to receive the *Miller Assessment for Preschoolers* (Miller 1988). Her parents and speech therapist were becoming increasingly concerned about her physical development.

Emily's mother reported that her pregnancy was uneventful. When Emily was born at full term, her birth weight was 4 lb. 13 oz. Shortly after birth, a congenital heart defect (atrial-septal defect) was discovered, but it was not severe enough to require surgery. She sat independently at 9 months, crawled at 11 months, and walked at 18 months. She began to feed herself at age 30 months. Her parents described her as withdrawn, shy, quiet, fearful, and anxious. She did not interact with other children. Her Miller Assessment results were all in the deficit range. For example, she was unable to localize which finger had been touched, put together a two-piece puzzle, differentiate simple figures from a background scene, or draw lines. Posturally, she was not able to stand with her feet together and close her eyes briefly, walk a tape line, imitate simple arm postures, or hold a supine flexion position (rounded into a ball holding forehead to knees while lying on her back).

Initially, Emily attended therapy sessions of 20 to 30 minutes three times per week. This schedule was suggested by her mother to help Emily become familiar with the clinic and the therapist. Gradually, Emily was able to participate in therapy activities without her mother's presence in the room. Activities were chosen to facilitate the development of muscle tone, muscle strength, movement procession (vestibular), accepting more textures (decreasing tactile defensiveness), and promoting body awareness. After approximately three weeks of therapy, her speech therapist reported a significant increase in Emily's spontaneous vocalizations. This is frequently seen in children who have vestibular processing deficits. As the vestibular system begins to process movement information, other parts of the brain also receive input.

At age 4, Emily entered a private school that specialized in working with children who have language deficits. The teachers at the school requested an inservice to explain the theories of sensorimotor and sensory integration therapies. The meeting provided an opportunity for sharing information. The teachers described certain techniques which they had found to be successful. The therapist was able to provide information about the sensory processing of the brain. This shared information assisted the teachers in defining educational goals and made the therapist more aware of her own therapy goals. A number of the teachers took a field trip to Emily's occupational therapy clinic to observe one of her sessions.

Emily received regular therapy for approximately 36 months. Her progress was slowing, and her parents felt they should concentrate more on Emily's language and learning delays. A favorite recollection of Emily and her family is the day her mother said, "Emily actually hugged me today! I know her muscle tone is improving because she has never hugged me before. You should have seen her daddy smile."

Case Study #6—Brady

Brady was referred for an occupational therapy evaluation by a family therapist who was working with his parents. They reported that he was extremely difficult for them to discipline. While his mother described him as a sweet and sensitive child, she found him to be extremely aggressive. He seemed particularly combative when his stepfather attempted to discipline him. He was prone to temper tantrums and crying spells. They had sought help from a family therapist when Brady was discovered taking knives from the kitchen and hiding them in his room.

The family therapist observed Brady with his parents, and found him to be extremely reactive to touch. She suggested that tactual defensiveness might be a problem for him, and recommended an occupational therapy evaluation to assess sensory integration.

The evaluation confirmed a finding of hypersensitivity to touch in addition to underresponsiveness to movement. Further testing could not be completed at the initial session due to Brady's extremely aversive response to the therapist's touch. He ran from the testing room and into the clinic, where he ran in circles for several minutes before he began kicking walls and throwing himself into therapy mats. The therapist was eventually able to calm him by providing deep-touch pressure in the therapy mats.

It was decided to begin therapy two times a week for one-hour sessions. In addition, the parents were to continue in their family therapy.

In early sessions, Brady sought out heavy work activities such as pushing against large therapy balls which were stabilized by the wall. This type of activity seemed to allow him to calm his overaroused nervous system. When he would tire from this activity, the therapist coaxed him into a suspended therapy net, where he requested to be pushed "faster and higher." He showed an extremely high tolerance for swinging and spinning, and soon began to seek out this activity without therapist direction.

In his first few weeks of therapy, he threw temper tantrums when his session was over and it was time to go. He screamed, cried, and hit, shouting, "I'm not leaving. You can't make me go." Eventually, he became able to tolerate leaving with the promise that he could come again soon.

Brady continued in therapy through the summer and began first grade in his public school in the fall. Shortly after beginning school, he began to receive "sad faces" for not completing his work. He showed poor attention and seemed immature as compared to his classmates. He was evaluated by the school psychologist, who felt that he showed an attention deficit disorder and referred him to his pediatrician for medication. The pediatrician decided not to prescribe medication at that point. She had observed a positive response to therapy, and recommended that Brady continue in his therapy program. She would reevaluate Brady's need for medication at a later time.

Brady continued to seek out intense movement and heavy work activities during therapy sessions. He also began to receive occupational therapy at school, which addressed visual-perceptual problems and helped his classroom teacher to respond more effectively to his behavior problems. The school therapist provided a large box with pillows in it where Brady was allowed to go for quiet time. This was used as a reward and not for punishment. The occupational therapist also encouraged his teacher not to keep him in from recess to finish his work, but instead to modify the amount of work so that he could succeed. Brady continued to respond well to his therapy program and developed a more positive attitude toward school.

Brady's family was provided with suggestions to support his therapy program. These included increased opportunities to meet his need for movement. They began to plan family outings to parks. His stepfather was advised to "play wrestle" with him, providing both movement and deep-touch pressure. His mother offered touch experiences such as clay-dough and shaving-cream play.

As Brady's sensory processing normalized, he was able to perform more successfully in the classroom. Gradually the teacher was able to increase the length of his assignments in response to his increased time on task. He was able to integrate into the classroom as his seating assignment was changed from a single desk set apart from the others to a desk in the front row. He moved from individual tasks to small-group work with other children. He was able to tolerate the noise and distractions of the cafeteria and the gymnasium.

By the time he entered second grade, Brady's behavior and school performance had improved significantly, but poor attention continued to be a problem. He began to take Ritalin and seemed to be in better control of his behavior both at home and at school. He continued in therapy privately and at school through the fourth grade. He remained on Ritalin through his elementary years. Now in junior high, Brady is a good student and plays trumpet in the band.

Case Study #7—Jonathan

Jonathan was referred for an occupational therapy evaluation on the recommendation of a hospital-based diagnostician. The diagnostician had been consulted by his mother when Jonathan was 7 years old because of poor coordination which his mother felt was related to a head trauma he had received at age 3. His medical history was significant for apnic (stoppage of breathing) episodes as an infant, asthma, and a history of ear infections that required two sets of pressure-equalizing tubes. His mother was concerned that he appeared clumsy as compared to other boys his age. She also reported possible visual-perception problems, poor handwriting, and poor task completion.

The diagnostician who saw Jonathan suggested that he might benefit from occupational therapy using sensory integrative techniques. The *Sensory Integration and Praxis Tests* indicated poor motor-planning abilities, touch sensitivity, and mild deficits in processing movement. He showed poorly established hand dominance which was felt to reflect poor communication between the two hemispheres of the brain. Jon was much heavier than his stepbrother and sister, which his mother attributed to limited physical activity due to his asthma.

Jon was screened for occupational therapy services through his public school, but did not qualify because his deficits did not appear to affect his classroom performance. Following private testing, it was recommended that he receive occupational therapy twice a week for 30-minute sessions. One of Jon's most notable traits was his extreme willingness to please. He worked very hard in his therapy program. The therapist continually challenged him to attempt new tasks. At first the challenges were fairly simple, such as asking him to climb a "mat mountain" composed of therapy mats. Soon he was able to climb the mountain and swing off, using a trapeze. Initially, he was able to ride a scooterboard down an inclined ramp, but not to pull himself back up the ramp. As he gained in strength, he began to pull himself up the ramp and to increase his speed and the number of repetitions.

Jon lived with his mother and stepfather, who were very supportive and encouraged him in academic skills, music, and drama. However, they did not encourage physical activity, believing that his medical history prevented him from pursuing even mild physical activity. The therapist encouraged them to begin a walking program and to encourage Jon to try a summer swimming program.

Jon had been in therapy for about six months when his natural father moved to town following discharge from the military. His father was a very physical man who complained that Jon had become a "Mama's boy." When Jon spent weekends with him, he would encourage morning runs and strenuous bike rides. He discounted the mother's concern for Jon's asthma and felt that Jon needed to "get tough," lose weight, and "shape up." His well-intentioned fitness program resulted in Jon's having a severe asthma attack that required hospitalization and ongoing respiratory therapy.

After Jon had regained sufficient health to resume his therapy program, his father consulted with the therapist. He asked about the nature and purpose of the therapy, stating that he did not communicate with Jon's mother and felt that she overprotected their son. After discussing the initial evaluation results, treatment plan, and Jon's success in therapy, his father became an advocate of his therapy program and frequently brought him for his sessions. He gradually learned to work within Jon's limitations and to be supportive of interests other than physical activities. He also encouraged Jon to become increasingly active, involving him in walking and recreational biking.

Over the course of his therapy, Jon lost weight, gained strength and endurance, and became increasingly confident of his newfound physical ability. He also improved in handwriting skills, organizational skills, and overall school performance. A positive side benefit was that his parents began to communicate. His father came to respect his mother's fears and to share her concerns for Jon's health. His mother came to trust his father's desire to help Jon become more physically active. They began to work together to support Jon in his therapy program and in his other endeavors.

Case Study #8—Sarah

Sarah was 5 years old when she was referred to occupational therapy by her school-district speech therapist. The speech therapist's evaluation revealed poor swallowing, garbled speech, drooling, and poor oral-motor function. She also noted generalized poor muscle tone. The school-district occupational therapist's test results were not within the range to qualify her for services. It was also noted that Sarah had superior academic abilities.

At the initial interview, Sarah's mother reported that she developed diabetes during her pregnancy with Sarah. Otherwise, her pregnancy and delivery were normal. Sarah had met her developmental milestones somewhat late (for example, walking at 17 months). At age 4, she had been examined by a neurologist, who diagnosed benign congenital hypotonia but identified no structural brain damage.

The occupational therapy evaluation consisted of administration of the *Sensory Integration and Praxis Tests* (Ayres 1989) in addition to clinical observations of eye and hand usage, postural responses, and other neuromuscular conditions relating to behavior and learning.

The evaluation identified deficits in vestibular processing, dyspraxia, tactual defensiveness, and poor gross motor and fine motor developmental. A treatment program was designed to address the identified deficits by providing vestibular and tactile stimulation, as tolerated; and gross motor and fine motor activities aimed at improving motor planning. Because of the severity of Sarah's problems, it was decided to provide two hours of private occupational therapy per week in addition to speech therapy provided through her public school.

During early sessions, it was apparent that strength and endurance were definite problems for Sarah. Although she always entered therapy eagerly, she fatigued quickly. Fortunately, her endurance increased; and definite gains were noted in both muscle strength and muscle tone.

During her sessions, she almost always gravitated toward intense vestibular activities, sitting or lying prone in a suspended therapy net and engaging in various activities such as throwing beanbags at a target.

Praxis (motor planning) was a definite problem area for Sarah, and it was felt that the praxis issues adversely affected her speech. The therapist incorporated oral-motor activities into the therapy sessions. For example, Sarah was encouraged to "paint" with her tongue, using pudding on a sheet of waxed paper. Another activity was using her tongue to push animal crackers from one side of a paper to another. When the goal was accomplished, she was allowed to eat the animal cracker.

Other more general activities were also used to address motor planning. Sarah was asked to maneuver a scooterboard through a course defined by cones. She was presented with suspended obstacle courses calling for transfers between pieces of therapy equipment such as bolsters, ladders, and inner tubes.

Sarah showed dramatic improvement in her motor skills and in her speech. One noticeable change was her newfound willingness to speak for herself. According to her mother, for years Sarah had allowed her sister (one year younger) to speak for her, particularly in the school setting. Sarah's assertiveness was a pleasant surprise to her parents, teachers, and classmates.

After one year of successful treatment, Sarah's parents were forced to withdraw her from therapy because their insurance carrier discontinued coverage. Unfortunately, the results were disastrous. Sarah soon began to lose ground with respect to her peers. While she maintained skills, the fatigue returned and caused her to withdraw from activities she had begun to enjoy. Her mother reported that she was too tired after a day at school to attend Girl Scout meetings. Her self-esteem began to suffer, and this recently outgoing, confident young lady became quiet and shy.

Because of the losses observed, her father took a second job in order to allow her to return to therapy. Sadly, an absence of six months cost her dearly in terms of the previous gains. The Bruininks-Oseretsky *Test of Motor Proficiency* (Bruininks 1978) showed that she had made no gains in the absence of therapy and had indeed lost ground in the areas of running speed and strength. Her original program was reinstated, and again she responded favorably. In addition to private therapy, she was determined to be eligible to receive occupational therapy services through her school program.

While her private program continued to focus on the identified deficits in vestibular and tactile processing and praxis, her school program focused specifically on educationally relevant activities such as visual-motor integration. Modifications included reduced written work, photocopies of boardwork to be used at her desk, and large-ruled paper for written assignments.

Over the course of her therapy, Sarah made significant gains in vestibular processing and associated gains in muscle tone. Her gross motor and fine motor skills improved, as did her ability to motor plan. While tactile defensiveness was addressed throughout the course of her therapy, extreme ticklishness remained a problem area for her, even at discharge. Along with the identified motoric gains, her speech showed dramatic improvement.

Sarah was discharged from occupational therapy at the age of 10. While she remained relatively frail in respect to her peers, she participated fully in physical education and in other activities such as Girl Scouting. She and her parents were very pleased with her abilities and with her eagerness to participate in both physical and socially appropriate activities.

In a recent phone call, her mother reported that Sarah, now 12, continues to do well. She is in resource classes at school and is making straight A's. She uses a keyboard at home and at school. Her favorite after-school activity is roller skating, and she is able to lace and tie her own skates.

References

Ayres, A. J. 1972. *Southern California sensory integration tests.* Los Angeles: Western Psychological Services.

_____. 1985. *Adult-onset apraxia and developmental dyspraxia.* Torrance, CA: Sensory Integration International.

_____. 1989. *Sensory integration and praxis tests.* Los Angeles: Western Psychological Services.

Beery, Keith E., and Norman A. Buktenica. 1989. *Developmental test of visual-motor integration.* Cleveland: Modern Curriculum Press.

Bruininks, Robert H. 1978. *Bruininks-Oseretsky test of motor proficiency.* Circle Pines, MN: American Guidance Service.

Cochran, C. 1986. Annotated bibliography: Vestibular-proprioceptive and tactile kinesthetic intervention for premature infants. *Physical and occupational therapy in pediatrics* 6(2):87.

DeGangi, G. A., and R. A. Berk. 1983. *Test of sensory integration.* Los Angeles: Western Psychological Services.

Dunn, Winnie. 1981. *A guide to testing clinical observations in kindergartners.* Rockville, MD: American Occupational Therapy Association.

Folio, M. R., and R. R. Fewell. 1983. *Peabody developmental motor scales and activity cards: Manual.* Allen, TX: DLM Teaching Resources.

Kimball, J. G. 1986. Prediction of methylphenidate (Ritalin) responsiveness through sensory integrative testing. *American Journal of Occupational Therapy* 40(4):241-48.

Miller, L. J. 1988. *Miller assessment for preschoolers.* San Antonio, TX: The Psychological Corporation.

Miller, L. J., S. H. Cohn, and P. Lemerand. 1988. Brief report: A summary of three predictive studies with the MAP. *Occupational Therapy Journal of Research* 7(6):378.

Riley, Glyndon D. 1972. *Riley motor problems inventory.* Los Angeles: Western Psychological Services.

Tupper, L. C. 1990. Richard: A case study employing the SIPT. *American Journal of Occupational Therapy* 44(7):647-49.

Wechsler, D. 1974. *Wechsler intelligence scale for children—Revised.* San Antonio, TX: The Psychological Corporation.

Wilbarger, P., and J. L. Wilbarger. 1991. *Sensory defensiveness in children aged 2-12.* Santa Barbara, CA: Avanti Educational Programs.

Wilson, Brenda. 1995. Use of the Bruininks-Oseretsky *Test of motor proficiency* in occupational therapy. *American Journal of Occupational Therapy* 49(1):8-17.

Readings—Sensory Integration and Sensory Systems

Ayres, A. J. 1972. *Sensory integration and learning disorders.* Los Angeles: Western Psychological Services.

_____. 1974. *The development of sensory integrative theory and practice.* Dubuque, IA: Kendall/Hunt Publishing.

_____. 1979. *Sensory integration and the child.* Los Angeles: Western Psychological Services.

Chusid, Joseph G. 1982. *Correlative neuroanatomy and functional neurology.* 18th ed. Los Altos, CA: Lange Medical Publications.

Clark, Ronald G. 1975. *Essentials of clinical neuroanatomy and neurophysiology.* Philadelphia: F. A. Davis.

deQuiros, Julio B., and N. L. Orland Schrager. 1979. *Neuropsychological fundamentals in learning disabilities.* Novato, CA: Academic Therapy Publications.

Fisher, Anne G., Elizabeth A. Murray, and Anita C. Bundy. 1991. *Sensory integration theory and practice.* Philadelphia: F. A. Davis.

Heiniger, Margot C., and Shirley L. Randolph. 1981. *Neurophysiological concepts in human behavior: The tree of learning.* St. Louis: C. V. Mosby.

Resource—Sensory Integration International

Sensory Integration International
P.O. Box 9013
Torrance, CA 90508
Telephone: 310-320-9986
FAX: 310-320-9934

Sensory Integration International is a nonprofit organization that encourages the exchange of information and expertise.